"Chris unfolds truths in this book that will set you on a path to healing and freedom only found in Jesus."

—DAVE AND ANN WILSON, hosts of *FamilyLife Today*

"The potency of Christopher's words will point you toward healing in your spirit, soul, and body. This journey of transformation isn't easy, but it's worth it."

—DANIEL G. AMEN, MD, psychiatrist and *New York Times* bestselling author

"This is a well-crafted, practical guide that will help you discover the courage to get up out of past trauma and follow the loving God who is constantly calling us forward."

—JAMIE WINSHIP, co-founder of the Identity Exchange and author of *Living Fearless*

"Chris compels us to move toward thoughtful daily rhythms that will transform our hearts, minds, and spirits. The words within this book strike a beautiful balance—they are both a balm for the hurting and a wake-up call for the brave."

—HANNAH BRENCHER, author of *Fighting Forward* and *Come Matter Here*

"This book is a pathway to life as God intended. It offers the insight you need to faithfully endure and overcome what you couldn't alter."

—DHARIUS DANIELS, author of *Relational Intelligence* and lead pastor of Change Church

"Chris has learned the necessity of transforming his deep pain into deeper perspective, power, and peace. He maps out the hope-filled path that led him to healing to help you get there as well. You may not be able to change your past, but you can certainly heal from it."

—DEBRA FILETA, MA, LPC, licensed counselor and bestselling author

"Christopher is a beautiful man with a deep heart for restoration in the lives of everyone he meets. I think you'll find this book immensely kind, gentle, and effective."

—JOHN ELDREDGE, bestselling author of *Wild at Heart* and *Resilient*

"Christopher Cook invites us all on a journey to the source of true healing. Although it requires walking through valleys we may believe we are not strong enough to walk through, he helps us to see we are not walking alone through Jesus."

—NONA JONES, speaker and author of *Killing Comparison*

healing
what
you can't
erase

healing
what
you can't
erase

Transform Your Mental, Emotional, and
Spiritual Health from the Inside Out

CHRISTOPHER COOK

FOREWORD BY DR. JOHN DELONY

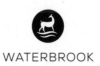

WATERBROOK

All Scripture quotations, unless otherwise indicated, are taken from the ESV® Bible (The Holy Bible, English Standard Version®), copyright © 2001 by Crossway, a publishing ministry of Good News Publishers. Used by permission. All rights reserved. Scripture quotations marked (AMPC) are taken from the Amplified® Bible, copyright © 1954, 1958, 1962, 1964, 1965, 1987 by the Lockman Foundation. Used by permission. (www.lockman.org). Scripture quotations marked (MSG) are taken from The Message, copyright © 1993, 2002, 2018 by Eugene H. Peterson. Used by permission of NavPress. All rights reserved. Represented by Tyndale House Publishers. Scripture quotations marked (NET) are taken from the NET Bible®, copyright © 1996, 2019 by Biblical Studies Press LLC (http://netbible.com). All rights reserved. Scripture quotations marked (NIV) are taken from the Holy Bible, New International Version®, NIV®. Copyright © 1973, 1978, 1984, 2011 by Biblica Inc.™ Used by permission of Zondervan. All rights reserved worldwide. (www.zondervan.com). The "NIV" and "New International Version" are trademarks registered in the United States Patent and Trademark Office by Biblica Inc.™ Scripture quotations marked (NKJV) are taken from the New King James Version®. Copyright © 1982 by Thomas Nelson. Used by permission. All rights reserved. Scripture quotations marked (NLT) are taken from the Holy Bible, New Living Translation, copyright © 1996, 2004, 2015 by Tyndale House Foundation. Used by permission of Tyndale House Publishers, Carol Stream, Illinois 60188. All rights reserved.

Italics in Scripture quotations reflect the author's added emphasis.

Names and minor details in some stories have been changed to protect the identities of the persons involved.

Library of Congress Cataloging-in-Publication Data
Names: Cook, Christopher (Pastor), author.
Title: Healing what you can't erase: transform your mental, emotional, and spiritual health from the inside out / Christopher Cook.
Description: First edition. | Colorado Springs: WaterBrook, 2024. | Includes bibliographical references.
Identifiers: LCCN 2023054132 | ISBN 9780593445303 (hardcover; acid-free paper) | ISBN 9780593445310 (ebook)
Subjects: LCSH: Spiritual healing. | Well-being—Religious aspects—Christianity.
Classification: LCC BT732.5 .C55 2024 | DDC 234/.131—dc23/eng/20240124
LC record available at https://lccn.loc.gov/2023054132

Printed in the United States of America on acid-free paper

waterbrookmultnomah.com

2 4 6 8 9 7 5 3 1

First Edition

Most WaterBrook books are available at special quantity discounts for bulk purchase for premiums, fundraising, and corporate and educational needs by organizations, churches, and businesses. Special books or book excerpts also can be created to fit specific needs. For details, contact specialmarketscms@penguinrandomhouse.com.

To you, my reader.
My fervent prayer is that the testimony of your life
will be marked by transformation and wholeness.
Take courage. Get up. He's calling you.

FOREWORD

I first met Christopher Cook at a private, invitation-only event in Nashville, Tennessee. There was a small group of new podcasters, YouTube stars, and public speakers, gathered from all over the country. The hotel conference room was full of money experts, a few mental health folks, a Navy SEAL, fitness gurus, pastors . . .

And me.

I was the dean of students at a university in Nashville, and I was considering making the seemingly insane leap of leaving my dream job to begin a career in media: from chief student affairs officer to, as my young son mocks me, YouTuber. I was an anxious fish out of water, because, although I pretend to be a loud and gregarious fun guy, I'm a closet introvert, always trying to cover up my insecurities and fears with more volume and relational sleight of hand.

I met many wonderful people that weekend, but one man in particular *saw through me:* Christopher Cook. Instead of being impressed and distracted by my dog and pony show, Chris cut through my anxiety and self-doubt, and he talked to me with interest, compassion, and powerful encouragement.

Chris spoke to me as someone who was on the Path. Someone who had been there. He knew something I didn't know: He was, in real time, healing, transforming, and growing into the person God was calling him to be. I didn't know his backstory or the extraordinary things he has endured and overcome. I didn't know about his work as a coach and pastor, or about his extraordinary podcast. I just knew he saw me clearly, and he encouraged me to jump.

Fast-forward several years and I'm reading the manuscript of the book you now hold in your hands. In the four short years since Chris and I first met, the world has changed dramatically. I'm looking across a burning landscape of political division, Covid-19, escalating global tensions, war, and fractured trust in the most essential pillars of society: church, education, medicine, and government.

We are living through a time when much of what we have taken for granted as wisdom or "right" is dissolving before our eyes. And while revealing falsehood is always a good thing, it is also unnerving when new truth isn't readily available to take its place. We all feel this anxiety.

Here are the facts: More people than ever are under the care of a licensed mental health professional, and more people than ever are taking some type of psychotropic medication. People in the United States are streaming out of the church. They are quiet quitting at work, and they are borrowing unprecedented amounts of money to prop up a fantasy lifestyle of comfort, indulgence, and survival. At the same time, people are increasingly more depressed, anxious, and frazzled. We are distracted, lonely, and Netflix-ing ourselves to death.

We have everything at our fingertips, and we've created a bronze statue of the Self and placed it in the center of the universe. And yet we're sick, divided, and awash in shame, anxiety, and depression.

Someone needs to call out the truth: What we're doing isn't working.

And like a phoenix rising from the ashes of a culture that has burned itself to the ground, Chris's book arrives on the scene, offering another way, a blueprint for moving into true healing, peace, and transformation.

As he did with me, Chris is staring a hole through the chaos, anger, and divisiveness. He reveals our God-less self-help culture for what it is: A fraud. A facade. A sham. A map to nowhere.

If self-help books truly did their job, we'd have a much different cultural, political, and relational zeitgeist. We'd have joy, laughter, and peace.

But we don't. We have chaos and disconnection instead.

We've been told that mental health is just getting all the right thoughts in just the right order. We destroy our bodies and our nervous systems for peace. We are told to forgive and forget, to "just get over" the traumas in our lives. Or worse, we're told that we will always be the worst things that ever happened to us. We spend our lives wallpapering over traumas, hurt, and grief with deep breathing exercises, politics, achievements, running away, or pseudo-religious performances.

And we find ourselves here. Tired, exhausted, and wanting to heal . . . but not knowing where to turn or whom to trust. Christopher Cook is just the author for such a time as this.

In *Healing What You Can't Erase*, Chris takes, head-on, the most terrifying questions of our time: *What if I can't fix myself, all by myself? What if I'm not good enough or strong enough to do it all, all by myself? How do I trust God when I've suffered and experienced life-altering pain and loss? If the self-help books are all wrong, what do I do now? How do I find peace?*

Chris is a coach, pastor, and podcaster, and in his book, he weaves a tapestry of theology, psychology, neuroscience, and his own incredible personal story to take us from a place of despair to action. From navel-gazing to submission. From shame, lack of trust, loss of identity, and trauma to a place of healing, transformation, and peace.

Chris gives us what most modern "how to heal" books lack: the truth. Things happen to us that simply cannot be erased. They are forever part of us. But they are not our destiny either. God is not calling us to a whitewashed life full of forgetfulness and ease. He's calling us into a messy new life, *especially* including what happened to us in our past. This life isn't about comfort; it's about peace.

If you're hurting, exhausted, lonely, and done with the cheesy five-step plans to wellness, a church that has left you for more smoke and lasers, or trying to be the center of your own universe, *Healing What You Can't Erase* is a cup of cold water for your weary soul. It is a blueprint for what to do next—a roadmap for a lost soul.

As you read, you'll feel Chris staring into you, as he did me at our fateful meeting years ago. You'll feel called out, yet encouraged, supported, educated, and loved—all powerful, right, and holy things. I have the privilege of calling Chris my friend, and though you may not know him personally, this book is the next best thing.

May the God of the universe bless you as you read. Over time, may you find peace. I promise it's real.

You can heal. You can be transformed. This book shows you how.

—Dr. John Delony, bestselling author, mental health expert,
and host of *The Dr. John Delony Show*

CONTENTS

START HERE

———————————

Healing what you can't erase. It's a deeply personal phrase I've been thinking about for the past decade. Not only does it describe the restoration I experienced after years of adversity and loss, but the implication therein is my greatest desire for you as we journey together through this book—that you, too, would receive physiological, mental, emotional, and spiritual healing from the pain-filled experiences that can never be erased from your life's story.

While I don't know the exact circumstances that brought us together on this page, there's a good chance that you might be feeling stuck or perhaps overwhelmed in a particular area of life right now. And as a result, you're languishing or in a state of depression or unrelenting anxiety—or you have some other form of psychological or emotional distress. Consequently, at some point along the way, you might have even thought, *I can't do this anymore,* or worse, *I don't want to do this anymore.* And if that's the case, I hope you don't interpret my words as being dismissive or callous when I tell you that I'm not surprised.

Multiple sources estimate that in the United States alone, forty million adults (those aged eighteen years and older) suffer from various anxiety disorders.[1] Of course, there's little doubt about the fact that the coronavirus pandemic that began in March 2020 enflamed many of these issues and pushed them into center stage of our cultural conversation. A Pew Research study revealed that "at least four-in-ten U.S. adults (41%) have experienced high levels of psychological distress at least once since the early stages of the coronavirus outbreak."[2] Remarkably, the same study said that "a 58% majority of those ages 18 to 29 have experienced high levels of psychological distress at least once across four Center surveys conducted between March 2020 and September 2022."[3] *Fifty-eight percent.* And as for post-traumatic stress disorder, the National Institutes of Health reports that "about 6 of every 10 men (or 60%) and 5 of every 10 women (or 50%) experience at least one trauma in their lives."[4]

That said, even though there is evidence of an uptick in depression, anxiety, and other mental and emotional health challenges within the last several years, the conditions themselves are nothing new to humanity. Centuries ago, the prophet Isaiah wrote, "Behold, darkness shall cover the earth, and thick darkness the peoples; but the LORD will arise upon you, and his glory will be seen upon you."[5] Darkness speaks of misery and sorrow.[6] One commentator explained, "*Darkness* constitutes both the circumstances of life and the experience of people."[7]

Sound familiar?

"But," he continued, "the solution lies in what happens to *you.*"[8]

And there's our key. Did you catch it? The solution is found in what happens *to you.* This is the work of transformation.

Healing what you can't erase doesn't mean ignoring the devastation of your past or putting a glossy spin on tragedy. That plastic version of faith isn't actually faith; it's immaturity and unbelief. Instead, healing what you can't erase is about moving forward through every loss, *scars and all,* while being transformed by the Holy Spirit's power toward wholeness in your physiology, your mental and emotional health, and your human spirit.

That's what this book is all about.

In the following pages, I'll share the candid details of my own story—as a precursor to unpacking the principles that forged my roadmap to wholeness. I must caution you, however, that the path we will tread together is neither the shortest nor the easiest. But the extent to which you accept the pain of change and growth will be the measure of healing you experience. That's not hyperbole either. That's the story of my life.

The principles you're about to learn aren't "five steps to live your best life." After all, what you hold in your hands is a roadmap, not a formula. As a pastor, a coach, and simply a person whose passion is *your* transformation, I'm here to guide you down a path that will be familiar to us both yet unique to you and your circumstances. Having said that, here's what you can expect:

In part 1, "The Breaking," you will learn that

- each day, we can all choose to say yes to participate in the process of transformation by the power of the Holy Spirit;
- while we can position ourselves for healing, we cannot turn the key to systemic transformation in life by our own determination, desire, or will; and
- healing a wounded, broken spirit is a linchpin for transformation.

In "The Building," part 2, you'll see why

- when shame enters our stories, what we tell ourselves is not based simply upon our actions but rather our inherent value as individuals;
- shame thrives in secrecy, often manifests in self-protection or self-promotion, and affects our spirits, souls, and bodies;
- the art of surrender is less about giving *up* and more about giving *in* to a process of confrontation that leads to life transformation from the inside out;
- entering the grief process is a necessary trek to help us eventually move forward in life;
- real peace is not a soul state absent of conflict;

- the output of our lives is wholly contingent on the interior health of our hearts;
- we are the ones who must take responsibility for our health and growth; and
- we must never underestimate the strength of our minds to steer our lives.

And part 3, "The Beckoning," will help you

- establish and fortify your true identity in Christ as your foundation stone of transformation.

At the end of each chapter, you'll find guided questions aimed at helping you personalize and assimilate your learnings. That's because life transformation requires consistent application. It is an ongoing work of the Holy Spirit, not a onetime event. So, as you set forth to heal what can't be erased, hear Isaiah's clarion call to you today:

Arise [from the depression and prostration in which circumstances have kept you—rise to a new life]! Shine (be radiant with the glory of the Lord), for your light has come, and the glory of the Lord has risen upon you![9]

Are you ready? Let's get started.

PART I

————

THE BREAKING

ONE

"HOLE"-NESS

Pain insists upon being attended to. God whispers to us
in our pleasures, speaks in our consciences, but shouts in
our pain: it is His megaphone to rouse a deaf world.

—C. S. LEWIS, *The Problem of Pain*

Think back to the day when *it* happened. What is *it*? Maybe the
ugly divorce. The cancer diagnosis. The far-too-early death of a
loved one. The betrayal of trust in a relationship. The indescrib-
able and unidentifiable weight of defeat that keeps you from moving forward in life. The slow and steady buzz of anxiety that has
been with you for so long that you wouldn't even recognize Monday morning without it. Waking up in physical pain for the ump-
teenth day in a row, exacerbated by fear and anxiety that cloud
your view of a hope-filled future . . . or perhaps, just for once, a
pain-free afternoon.

Or how about the chatterbox of taunts that greet you every
morning before your feet hit the floor? *You talk too much. You're
not taken seriously. You're too sensitive. You're too needy. You're never
going to heal, so you might as well give up now. Your spouse is going
to cheat on you. Your children are in constant danger. It's too late. No
one really wants to be your friend. You're not good enough. You don't
have what it takes.*

It's tormenting, isn't it? For a lot of us, we are languishing, and anxiety, overwhelm, exhaustion, and cynicism are the norm, even though their presence in our lives is anything but normal. And the scariest part? We've endured those feelings and internal indictments for so long that we don't even know when they first showed up on our doorsteps.

That was my story.

The details I'm about to share are as raw as they are honest. But I'm beginning our relationship here because I want you to know right off the bat that you aren't alone in your pain and loss, even though I'm sure it feels like you are. I also realize that it's hard to step into someone else's trauma while walking through your own. And for that reason, I want to reassure you that, as you go through this book, you won't walk alone as you chart your path to wholeness either—the wholeness available only through the ongoing process of transformation by the power of the Holy Spirit at work within us. I pray that you'll learn from my experiences in both pain and healing. No doubt, I have plenty of scars. I'm sure you do too. But those scars tell a very personal story. And *that* story begins right now.

THE NIGHTMARE ON OUR STREET

Autumn had settled on the Midwest, and despite our reputation for brutal winters, this time of year was absolutely breathtaking. It was Saturday, November 3, 2012, and at a glance, you'd think it was going to be a picture-perfect day. Though the morning temperature was in the low forties, the sun was rising on the dew-covered grass, and the crisp air seemed to awaken the neighborhood in unison. Our family's quaint quad-level home, where we had lived for seventeen years, sat on the corner lot. Within its walls, Mom and Pops had hosted high school graduation parties, birthday celebrations, Thanksgiving dinners, and memorable get-togethers. And in the home office where my parents operated their professional counseling practice with precious care, marriages had been restored and many lives—young and old—given focus, compassion, challenge, and empowerment. To this day, when I envision a place of peace and rest, it's that house. The literal blood, sweat, tears, laughs, and sacrifices that built and rebuilt that house from the inside out made it our haven. It wasn't elaborate by any stretch, nor was it perfect, but it was perfectly ours.

Just across the street on that November morning, the sun's reflection shone on the tiny lake. The fiery colors of autumn blanketed the trees in the background. Trust me when I tell you that you haven't seen beauty until you've been to Michigan in the fall. If you don't believe me, book a trip here and witness it for yourself.

As I stepped off our front porch to go for a quick walk, our neighbor Lynn, with coffee in hand, sauntered to the edge of her driveway to retrieve the newspaper and waved in my direction. "Morning, Chris!" she exclaimed.

Have you ever been so deep in thought that you don't even hear someone talking to you? This was one of those times.

"Chris! Mornin', honey," she called in her soft, quintessential midwestern tone.

I waved back. "Morning, Lynn. Hope you and Tom have a good day." Truth be told, I wasn't lost inside my mind. I was *drowning* there. Allow me to explain.

That particular Saturday was my birthday, and it became the third-worst day of my life. You see, four weeks earlier, doctors had sent my mom home without any further medical recourse. At the age of fifty-five, she was fighting for her life after a nearly two-decade battle with multiple myeloma, a rare, medically incurable form of cancer. With tears in her eyes, my mom's oncologist placed her into hospice care—the very organization for which Mom was once the bereavement coordinator. If you're unfamiliar, when someone is placed on hospice, death has been declared imminent.

Despite this prognosis, our family was relentless in our pursuit of healing. Sobered by the medical facts, we were equally anchored in and focused on the truth of the Scriptures: Our God is a healer. We were tired, but we weren't giving up hope for a miracle. People had told us to stop playing "the faith game" and instead face the facts. But this was no game.

Through weeks of sleepless nights and tear-filled days, we poured ourselves into her care, often ignoring our own needs to provide for her in the most personal and intimate ways while protecting her dignity. Because Pops—hero that he is—worked three jobs for nearly twenty years to keep the family out of medical debt, my sister and I were on rotation, sleeping in our parents' bed to cover the arduous night shift with Mom. Our love was stronger than any embarrassment or shame at her total dependency, because her worth, value, dignity, and beauty were not clouded by the terrible disease destroying her outer shell.

Though Mom could barely speak or even keep her eyes open, multiple myeloma was not her identity. *She* was not cancer. And that's why I was internally distracted when Lynn called my name that morning. I was hoping that when I got home from my walk, somehow life would be good again. That all of this would be a bad dream. But it wasn't. I hated that day. I *hated* my birthday.

When I returned fifteen or twenty minutes later, I went upstairs to tend to Mom, who was barely conscious. I asked her, "Momma, do you know what today is?" She shook her head no. "It's my birthday! Do you know how old I am today?"

She whimpered, "A hundred and thirty-five?"

She wasn't trying to be playful, though her gregarious Italian personality, now absent, was my favorite part about her. She was in and out of a comatose state. I kissed her on the cheek and left the room for a moment, heading toward the bathroom as a flood of tears fell down my cheeks. I leaned into the sink and dropped my head. *How can this be real?* I turned on the faucet and splashed some cool water on my face.

That night, my sister and a few close friends took me to my favorite sushi restaurant for dinner. They sang "Happy Birthday," but I didn't hear anything. I could barely stomach my food. When I caught my sister's eyes a few times during the meal, I noticed she lifted a soft smile toward me, but I saw the shared exhaustion in her countenance.

THE STORM WE NEVER SAW COMING

Though this was the darkest chapter, our story began more than eighteen years prior on Monday, September 26, 1994—the *second*-worst day of my life. It was an unseasonably balmy day, the dark clouds were low, and the smell of an impending rainstorm was in the air.

Little did I know as an eleven-year-old seventh grader, though, that a storm more devastating than the lightning and thunder headed our way was about to upend our family's simple life. It was odd that Mom *and* Pops picked us up from school that day. Something was up.

After just a couple of minutes hearing about our days, they looked at each other and then Mom looked back at us. "I have cancer," she said. "But it's sleeping right now. We're going to be okay." Indolent multiple myeloma was the diagnosis, asymptomatic for the time being.

Doctors had never seen this disease in a thirty-seven-year-old Caucasian woman. She was an anomaly to say the least—one of the first Americans fitting that profile to be handed this diagnosis. At the time, my parents were told that myeloma typically showed up in elderly Black *men*.[1] Myeloma tends to be much more aggressive in younger patients too.[2] Not knowing exactly what to do, the doctors at a large hospital in Detroit had offered her two options: (1) a stem cell treatment that might buy her anywhere from six months to two years, or (2) do *nothing*.

With cries for help to the Lord, our family knelt together in prayer by the peach-colored camelback couch in the living room. I remember not sleeping well that night, and though I was nearing my twelfth birthday, I dug out my old Glo Worm nightlight and plugged it into the wall beside my bed. Yet not even that familiar soft glow could take away the fear of the dark so deep in my young soul.

The next day at school, my mom, like the poised and attentive counselor she was, met with my sister's and my teachers to let them know what was going on so they could provide a watchful eye over our temperaments and emotional dispositions through-out the day. Over the next several years, we adjusted to our family's new way of life. Cancer ebbed and flowed through everyday conversations most days.

Amid these pressing challenges, however, my sister and I had an incredible childhood. We had the best parents. Truly. They sacrificed a lot and worked multiple jobs to make sure we received a meaningful and impactful education. Our homelife was safe, stable, and nurturing. But the best part about growing up was our church friends. Not only were they our *best* friends, but they'd also become family and stood by us when we needed them most.

Eleven years into this fight against cancer, we finally felt like we were regaining a sense of routine . . . and hope. As a family, we eagerly anticipated good days ahead. Sadly, however, our expectations were shattered one afternoon in September 2005. As my mom opened the sliding glass door to let our dogs outside to play, a bee flew into the house and landed high on the kitchen window. Because my mom was severely allergic to bees, she quickly grabbed a fly swatter and lifted herself halfway up on the countertop to get a good swing. In the process, she overextended her back to such an extent that a loud popping sound, immediately followed by debilitating pain, ripped through her spine. Collapsing on the floor, she cried out for help. For the next seven months, Mom experienced a level of pain she had never known. Her surgeon diagnosed it as severely strained discs in the lumbar region of her spine.

FROM BAD TO WORSE

Soon after, things turned from a bad dream to a *nightmare*. On Monday, May 1, 2006, I walked up the sidewalk after a stressful day of work. Head down, I was already thinking about the paper I had to finish for one of my undergrad classes. Then I looked up toward the front door. Mom stood, frozen, on the other side of the glass. I nearly jumped backward. The color had drained from her face, and as soon as I opened the door, she threw the phone down, screamed, and fell into my arms. "There's cancer all over my body!" she cried.

An MRI had revealed that rather than displaced discs, her spine was full of bone marrow disease. The cancer was spreading. Had we not acted quickly, doctors speculated that with her stage IV disease progression, she might not have lived another thirty days.

Within an hour, our house was filled with our closest friends, pastors, and extended family. Shocked and stricken by grief and fear, I disappeared into the backyard alone, where I sat on the grass, paralyzed in terror. I didn't speak. I *couldn't* speak. I honestly don't remember much else about that day. Maybe that's from the trauma. But after an hour or so, my pastor came to sit with me. He had known me since I was a little boy, and I trusted him. His gentle presence told me that I was safe. All the pain I had evidently buried after Mom's original diagnosis rushed to the surface, and I wept in his arms. He just held me.

Two days later, we met with Mom's new local oncologist, who would soon launch a barrage of chemotherapy into her body to hold back the stampede of cancerous lesions quickly multiplying throughout her spine.

Over the next few years, there were more bad days than good. Don't get me wrong. We did experience good days, but they were almost always short-lived. It was like every good report came with a proverbial asterisk tacked on the end. In fact, when the phone rang at home, it was usually bad news from the doctor. Before long, the sound of the phone ringer itself—no matter *who* was calling—triggered panic that rushed through my nervous system. As you might expect, "on edge" became my normal state. I cried often. Depending on the day, the tears were an overflow of feeling exhausted, fearful, or inescapably trapped. Or a combination of all three.

You see, before I knew anything about wholeness, I encountered "hole"-ness: a soul state in which blistering divots caused by acute fearful, shame-filled experiences motivated me to hide inside myself, even while I wore the costumes of a smile and an upbeat personality. I'm not at all insinuating that I was living insincerely. I just didn't know where to slot the trauma responses, incessant chatter, and anxiety-ridden rumination that had been inside my head since childhood.

From 2006 to 2010, Mom was in and out of the hospital several times for various emergency surgeries and procedures. And then in mid-February 2011, on a snowy Thursday night, we had to call an ambulance because she couldn't move. She had a new tumor the size of a softball on her spine. The pain was unbearable. As snow fell on her frail body, the EMS workers carefully yet expeditiously wheeled her into the ambulance. Then Pops, in haste, fell down the stairs and broke his ankle just twenty minutes after the ambulance raced Mom to the hospital.

Two days later, we almost lost her in surgery. The rest of 2011 was a blur, but we still held on to hope for a miracle for Mom.

As I mentioned earlier, by the first week of October 2012, the medical community could offer no further assistance, and hospice care was called in. The night the hospice workers came to meet with my parents, I hid in my bedroom and shook violently as chills ran through my body. I sat on the floor, barely deciphering the details of the conversation taking place downstairs in the living room. I vaguely remember hearing a few questions: "With which funeral home should we coordinate your details?" and "Are your desires written in a will yet?" For the first time in almost eighteen years, I felt betrayed within the four walls of the safest place I had known throughout this storm: my home.

I'm sure that in your own story, you encountered an inflection point in which you realized there was no going back to normal—a point when even the most familiar parts of your life no longer felt like home. This was that night for me.

The following six weeks, October through mid-November, were the most devastating of all. Many nights, we were wide awake with Mom as she declined to a childlike, unrecognizable state. My sister and I had to frequently call the twenty-four-hour hospice care phone line for direction and assistance as the side effects of the medications prescribed for Mom's palliative care caused her to become belligerent. Those nights scared me. Where did my *mom* go?

As I already shared, my birthday came and went, and we were in the heat of the battle. There was no letting up. The lack of sleep took a toll on our bodies and minds. And though the calendar indicated that the holiday season was upon us, it meant nothing, for we were under siege. The explosion of autumn's colors painted a backdrop for absolute horror to unfold in the most devastating and unpredictable manner.

Then Wednesday, November 21, 2012, arrived: the *worst* day of my life.

At 11:40 A.M., my phone rang while I was at work. It was Carmen, my sister. In an unforgettable tone, she ordered, "Get home *now*. Mom stopped breathing." And like that . . . it was over. An eighteen-year battle. Over. I raced home, only to find her lifeless body. *Why didn't I get to say goodbye?* Apparently, she was still breathing until she was alone in her room, literally for a minute. Then she left.

What happened in the hours following was like punctuation on a sentence I never wanted spoken. I felt completely stripped and robbed, blindsided, and abandoned. Within an hour, the house was flooded with people. My extended family, our closest church friends, and others came to be with us. Some people attempted to offer "explanations" of the situation to invoke faith and trust, but I wanted none of it. It's not that they were insincere; I just wanted my mom back.

And like I did six years prior, I retreated to the backyard and stayed there for a couple of hours. I begged a friend to tell me when the funeral home had taken my mom's body away. I couldn't watch that scene unfold. Certainly, *that* would not be the final image of my mom forever painted on my heart. Later that night, all I remember is collapsing on our wooden stairs, battle-weary, as an uncontrollable flood of tears literally discolored a single plank of wood beneath me. When the cries of family members and friends joining us in our grief subsided, a deafening silence engulfed the house.

The next day, Thursday, was Thanksgiving. I stayed in my bedroom the whole day. Some family members came over with a turkey. Though there were no intentions of celebrating that day, they just wanted to be together. But what did I have to be thankful for? Oh, that even though Mom was gone, she was "in a better place"? Whatever. That she had "won"? *Who* won? All I knew was that even though Mom was in heaven, her absence hurt like hell.

Christmas 2012 came and went. Just a week later, 2013 arrived, and we were surviving. I barely spoke for two months after my mom died, and when I did, my words were few. As 2013 progressed, there were a few good days. Some days it felt like we were breathing again, though for the majority, it felt like we had been thrown back into a pit of despair. But that's grief. It's hardly tidy and linear. We'll talk about grief later in the book, but for now, I'll say this: Grief is like a wild river—it's unpredictable and messy. You probably know how this feels from times of loss and bereavement in your life. And while I'm not sure we ever get *over* grief, we do go *through* it.

That summer, Carmen got married. It was a beautiful day, yet it was marked with a keen presence of sadness. There was an empty chair in the front row, occupied only by a single sunflower. That was Mom's seat.

HIT WHILE I WAS DOWN

You know how it is when you've hit rock bottom and you think things can't possibly get worse? And then you realize they can? Yeah, me too. A few weeks later, on a humid Michigan morning in late-August 2013, I woke up and began my daily routine: make the bed, open the window blinds, head to the bathroom to insert my contact lenses. But when I put the contact lens in my right eye, something was off—my vision in that eye was slightly distorted. Convinced that the humidity and heat were simply exacerbating my allergies, especially in a house that lacked central air-conditioning, I took an antihistamine and went about my day.

But by late afternoon, the issue hadn't resolved. I called my doctor, who, luckily, squeezed me into his schedule late in the day. Upon investigation, he was puzzled and, truth be told, a little concerned. He arranged for me to see an ophthalmologist the next day. The ophthalmologist, a wonderful man, was gracious and very careful, but he, too, was concerned. Finally, after a battery of tests, he looked at me and said, "Internuclear ophthalmoplegia. Christopher, I need to call a neurologist and set up an appointment for you."

By September 2013, after another round of tests, a handful of appointments with specialists, and an MRI of my brain—*and* living through nearly a year of unrelenting post-traumatic stress, sleepless nights, and an unmanaged thought life fueled by the spirit of fear—my body couldn't withstand the internal battle any longer. Especially after this latest fiasco with my eye.

So, it broke. My body broke.

My immune system crashed in a nosedive that I never saw coming, especially because of the cloud of grief surrounding me. And so, on September 20, 2013, I sat in a neurologist's office, already in a fog of depression and anxiety, as he told me I had been diagnosed with a medically incurable autoimmune disease: relapsing-remitting multiple sclerosis (MS). Though he assured me that unlike the report given to many across the nation, my case was manageable and nonthreatening to my long-term livelihood, I was devastated.

Carmen came to the appointment with me. With poise and grace, she took notes and asked the questions I didn't even begin to know how to ask. Keep in mind, we weren't even a year into grieving the loss of our mom. I felt kicked and bruised while I was already down-and-out.

In the days and weeks following my diagnosis, I scoured the internet for case studies and anecdotal evidence of MS patients' success with various nutritional protocols. A repeated theme began to emerge: the efficacy of functional medicine principles combined with an anti-inflammatory Paleo diet and high-dose vitamin D_3, among other things. The repeated anecdotal evidence confirmed the direction I wanted to take in conjunction with classical therapies prescribed by my neurologist.

By late autumn of 2013, I sensed a glimmer of hope for life again as I settled into my new rhythm. Sadly, however, it was short-lived. As the holiday season approached, along with the one-year anniversary of Mom's passing, I could feel a blanket of heaviness hovering over my soul. The intensity of grief and our awareness of the permanence of our losses sure seem to dial up during the holidays, don't they?

I spent Christmas Day in bed. Not only was I in physical pain, but a cloud of depression and hopelessness like I had never known also arrived. Underneath the covers of my bed, I stared across my bedroom as tears filled my eyes. These tears were different, however. They didn't flow easily but instead dropped slowly and heavily. The exhaustion of the last year, particularly the final six weeks with my mom, and my own medical diagnosis left me battle-weary and defeated. Like many others who experience similar seasons of trauma, I didn't want to live. I never considered acting on that thought, but the profundity and severity of my broken spirit caught up with me in a frightening way.

As the new year arrived, I was going backward, even though I feigned a smile for almost everyone else. Why I did that, I don't know. I think I just didn't want to be burdensome to anyone. Have you ever felt that way? You rationalize that it is easier and less exhausting to avoid long conversations, and "I'm okay" becomes the de facto response to anyone who asks how you're doing.

And sure, I was following my treatment protocol, but the turmoil from within was hampering my body's ability to heal. Irrational fears from childhood reemerged in my heart, and I spiraled into obsessive-compulsive panic-stricken hypochondria on top of severe depression and anxiety. Every cluster headache and muscle spasm, every blood test and routine checkup with my neurologist thrust me into severe panic. All of this later led to a diagnosis of complex post-traumatic stress disorder.

And even though I received incredible support from my immediate family (who were grieving themselves) and close friends, there was only one person I wanted to talk to about my pain and my fears—my mom. Why, in the middle of our deepest pain, does it feel like the person we need most is the one who is gone?

Each morning, I awoke with tears in my eyes. I spent my lunch breaks at work sleeping, after setting my phone's alarm for twenty-five minutes in hope of giving my soul just a few moments of rest.

In March 2014, after more research for local medical support, I became a patient of a well-respected functional medicine doctor, formerly the head of internal medicine at a university hospital. During my intake appointment, my words were labored. I sat across from the doctor and wept. I didn't know how to ask for help anymore, let alone know what I needed in the first place. Frankly, I just wanted to find rest for my broken heart. Sensing my profound and immediate need, she momentarily hurdled the typical professional boundary between physician and patient. With great compassion, she rose from her desk, walked to the chair where I sat sunken in pain, and embraced me like a mom would her son. Though I was a grown adult, in that moment I felt like a little boy, desperate for help and safety. A torrent of emotion overcame me. With desperation and a whimper, I begged her to promise I would be okay. This was "hole"-ness at full tilt.

By the time springtime fully arrived, I had adjusted to the changes in my treatment protocol and felt more secure having a small team of professionals nearby. But the anxiety didn't let up. Each day, I was arrested by no fewer than twenty attacks. Thankfully, however, I learned how to breathe and move through each bout within a few minutes after their onset. Still, it felt like post-traumatic stress had latched on to my mind and body with no plans of letting go.

To cope, I created a very small, safe, but stuck existence. And though I had discovered a newfound love for running on the local junior high school track where my mom used to run when Carmen and I were kids, I rarely went anywhere outside a five-mile radius, and I *never* deviated from my routine.

As a very disciplined and structured person by nature, when I became overextended and stressed, I let structure become my source of stability. That's because the motivating fear in my life wasn't so much the fear of bad news but the fear of losing more control. And even though the predictability of my weekly routine gave me a refreshing taste of reprieve, I was stuck. Time was moving on, but I wasn't moving forward. Grief was no longer a process; instead, it became complicated. More often than not, I saw life through the lens of "what was" rather than "what is" and "what could be."

> The motivating fear in my life wasn't so much the fear of bad news but the fear of losing more control.

Being aware of my condition created more anxiety for my type A personality, but I really believe the Lord was waking me up to what was at stake. My pain was real. The trauma was legitimate. The losses were great. No one could deny that. But equally real was the existence of my purpose—a purpose I could have chosen to forsake. Something had to change.

SOMETHING HAD TO CHANGE

One Saturday night in late October 2014, I was home alone watching a basketball game on television. Unsettled by a nagging desire for something to change, I turned off the game and prayed.

Despite the pain and losses I'd endured, I still loved the Lord. Did I doubt Him? Of course. I was profusely mad at Him and felt betrayed when my mom died. And when my health collapsed shortly thereafter, I felt defeated and abandoned. But somehow, I never painted Him into a corner or staked the totality of my faith on one answer to prayer. Honestly, I attribute that posture to my mom. When Carmen and I were growing up, she would often share two foundational truths with us: "Nothing is impossible with the Lord" and "He is eternally good."

"Like a puppy on a leash," she'd say, "stay anchored in the goodness of God. Don't get too far removed from it, because if you do, you'll get bitter. And bitterness will kill you from the inside out." She was right.

My moment in prayer wasn't profound. I was tired and annoyed, and I just needed answers. "Lord, I can't live like this anymore," I stated matter-of-factly. "You have to do something. Heal me tonight. Please. I'm done. I don't know what, but *something* has to happen." That was it. I opened my eyes and sat on the couch in silence for a few minutes before turning the TV back on. I knew He heard my prayer and hoped that maybe by morning, something would change.

But then He spoke.

I knew it was Him because ever since I was a little boy, I had grown familiar with His still, small voice. It was an uncontested, undeniable knowing. But He didn't respond with "I see you. You're right. You're healed." Instead, He asked me a question: "What do you want Me to do for you?"

I knew immediately that I'd been set up. He wasn't asking me that question because He didn't know what I needed (or wanted). God is omniscient. He knows every word I will speak before I utter it. Instead, He was asking me a rhetorical question: Was I willing to take responsibility for my life and no longer find sufficiency in my deficiencies? Was I unwilling to allow one season, though long and painful, to write the whole story of my life? And while I couldn't turn the key on manifesting healing in any area of my life (He alone is healer), would I partner with Him and position myself for it?

It is the same question He asks you today. I don't believe you picked up this book by accident. If you're exhausted, confused, defeated, jaded, and hopeless, I see you. I'm so sorry for what happened. But just as He did for me, He's asking you, "What do you want Me to do for you?"

Within that question is an invitation to partner with the Lord in your own process of transformation. Trust me when I tell you that it won't happen in one day; it will be *daily*. Will change hurt? Yes. But the consequences of *not* changing are much greater, especially in the long run. Is healing costly? In more ways than one.

In fact, it might even seem like things get worse before they get better. But is transformation worth it? Is a life marked by wholeness far greater than the cost? Believe me when I say, unequivocally and assuredly, yes, it is. So lean in, and let's get started on transforming your mental, emotional, and spiritual health from the inside out.

PERSONALIZE IT

THE POINT

We all have the opportunity to participate in the daily process of transformation by the power of the Holy Spirit.

THE PROMPT

What do you want the Lord to do for *you*? Your answer might relate to a specific defining moment of crisis, loss, or disappointment (when *it* happened). And while your answer is valid, please remember that in my case, what I needed more than a change of circumstance was a change of heart. The Lord knew I wanted my circumstances to change. But His rhetorical question provoked me to get beyond the surface-level issue to the *deeper* one. And I believe the same will be true for you. This is the work of transformation.

THE POSTURE

Don't rush this very important first step. Before moving on, take ample time to gain clarity about the area(s) for which you desire transformation, as well as areas the Lord is leading you to confront and heal. And when you've painted a mental picture of what this looks like, I'll meet you in chapter 2.

THE PRAYER

Lord, I want to change. I want to experience healing for what can't be erased. So today, I say yes to Your invitation to transformation. I say yes to taking responsibility for my life. I give You access to my heart. Search me. Shape me. Sharpen me. It's for Your glory that I ask these things. Amen.

TWO

YOU ARE NOT ENOUGH

I have been driven many times upon my knees by the
overwhelming conviction that I had nowhere else to go.
My own wisdom and that of all about me seemed
insufficient for that day.

—PRESIDENT ABRAHAM LINCOLN

Had you and I met at a coffee shop a handful of years ago, a
few minutes into the conversation and a few sips into the coffee
(tea for me), you'd likely have asked me about the pristine black
D-ring binder nestled at my side. Arrayed with color-coded tabs
that separated hundreds of pages, it traveled with me wherever I
went. It was my escape plan—well, maybe not so much *escape* as
it was my seemingly bulletproof plan to get free and healthy again.
I'd relish the opportunity to proudly show you how I'd designed
the first three hours of every morning, contending that depression
and anxiety were done holding me hostage. A few pages in, I'd
show off my meal plans for the week, specific to the nutritional
value that research revealed would bring healing to my body. On
paper, it was flawless. But then you'd probably ask me how it was
going. And I'd change the subject. Because it wasn't.

It had been a few months since I heard the Lord ask me the
question "What do you want Me to do for you?" And though I
knew it was a rhetorical question about my willingness to take
responsibility for my life, I was already frustrated that my best

efforts to effect change in my life continued to come up short. Worse, everything I thought would be helpful—like getting regular counseling, changing my daily routine, and even overhauling my diet—was proving to be otherwise. I was confused. There was no doubt about what I wanted: freedom and healing. I had formulated a plan to make it happen, even with professional help. But why wasn't the plan working? Why did it seem like I was spinning my wheels? *Is it the grief? Is it depression? Or is all this a pipe dream?*

Suffice it to say, the burgeoning sense of overwhelm and defeat was intimidating, especially because I have always been a driven, disciplined person. Once I set my heart on something, I don't quit. In fact, that tenacity is what fanned the flames of unswerving dedication to my mom's physical care. But maybe that same drive had backfired on my body when trauma hit. All I know is that because of my failure to make this plan work, anxiety and depression flared up afresh. In those moments, I considered that after all I had been through, a small, stuck life was not only safe but perhaps even appealing.

Something had to change. But deep down, I knew that something was me. *I* had to change. Therein was the hurdle, however. I had the will (the desire and intention) but not the power to do so. No matter how hard I planned and worked, no amount of drive or determination seemed to turn the key on the transformation for which I was so desperate.

I'm sure you can relate. How often recently have you found yourself in a challenging situation for which you have a plan but, despite your best efforts, continue to come up short? As with me, it might be an overhaul of your health. But it could certainly involve breaking an old harmful habit, installing a new healthy habit, maturing in a relationship, or getting started on the project you've been putting off for far too long.

In the past year, I've endeavored to dig deeper to understand why we continue to hit the proverbial brick wall in this exact domain. After all, logic says, "Set your intention, develop a plan, and then get to work." It's straightforward advice, right? And even though much of the self-help industry hangs its hat on this formula,[1] why aren't the results consistent across the board? I believe the problem is not in the formula but in the means and motivation by which we execute the formula.

Consider this: Popular psychology preaches, "You are enough," but are you? Am I? Honestly, I don't think we are. You may have just bristled, but stay with me. What I'm exploring in *this* context is not our inherent value as ascribed by a loving God but our wherewithal, if any, to effect meaningful, sustainable transformation in our own lives. Left to our own agency, can we turn the key to unlock self-healing? Can we hurdle obstacles, narratives, and false identities that so easily strangle our potential and squander our years?

Well, according to the self-help industry's playbook, yes, we can. But why, then, are the outcomes so inconsistent? Is willpower reliable over time and even under stress? And worse, why do we keep repeating the same patterns even though the results don't typically validate our efforts? One psychologist has argued that it's how we're wired.

WILLPOWER, STRESS, AND OUR PHYSIOLOGY

"Focusing on the end result," Dr. Loyd wrote, "comes from your hardwired programming, otherwise known as your stimulus/response or seek pleasure/avoid pain programming. It's part of your survival instinct, and it's what you used almost exclusively during the first six or eight years of your life: want ice cream cone, plan to get ice cream cone, go get ice cream cone. That's why it feels so natural. The big problem is that as adults, we're not supposed to live this way unless our life is in immediate danger."[2] He believes that another reason we repeat the playbook's pattern (set your intention, create a plan, and then act on the plan) is that we have seen it repeated in nearly every context of personal growth and self-help.[3] And while the jury is still out on the substantive nature and capacity of willpower, that's not the basis for my argument here.

Scientists and psychologists have spent years discussing will-power as it relates to self-regulation and ego depletion (a hotly debated topic that some believe is a myth), as well as how our beliefs about its capacity affect our minds. But at the end of the day, my personal experience tells me that everyone will eventually run out of willpower because no one has unlimited capacity or supply.

Think about this: A sixteen-ounce water bottle and a five-gallon bucket have *different* but not *unlimited* capacities. And like those containers, each one of us has varying degrees of intellectual, emotional, and physical ability, but we are not without limit. Thus, as helpful as willpower might be to get us on the road, I don't believe it has the ability to get us to our desired destinations.

> As helpful as willpower might be to get us on the road, I don't believe it has the ability to get us to our desired destinations.

But for a moment, I want to take a step backward and ask you—especially if you're facing a signifi-cant challenge (or desire)—what do you *really* want? Here's what I mean: In my case, my black binder represented a written plan of action to get healthy again. But below the surface, what I *really* wanted was to know peace and hope and perhaps even regain a sense of self-confidence that had been buried by loss. Most of all, I wanted control of the life that had spun painfully outside of my control. With near-maniacal fervor, I wanted to wrap my arms so tightly around my life that no more damage could be incurred. I had been through enough, I thought, and I just wanted my life back, whatever that meant. But look carefully at my motivation. Was it based in rest and trust? Faith, hope, and love? No. I was motivated by fear, which put me in a cycle of chronic stress, caus-ing my nervous system to be stuck in a state of dysregulation.

Now, can fear be healthy to a degree? Can stress be beneficial? Of course. Not all stress is bad. Our bodies are capable of endur-ing stress in short bursts. Under imminent danger, fear and stress stimulate adrenaline, which aids our survival. In this state of fight or flight, the body shifts its resources to fending off an imminent threat or enemy, even if the "enemy" is inside our minds.[4] This is why we've heard stories of people performing dramatic feats to prevent danger or save a loved one.

"'Good stress,'" as defined by neuroendocrinologist Bruce McEwen, "refers to the experience of rising to a challenge, taking a risk and feeling rewarded by an often positive outcome."[5] We experience this kind of stress when we set meaningful goals, ask someone on a date and risk rejection, or leave a comfortable but mundane job for the uncertainty of a dream job.

"'Tolerable stress,'" on the other hand, "refers to those situations where bad things happen, but the individual with healthy brain architecture is able to cope, often with the support of family, friends and other individuals. These adverse outcomes can be 'growth experiences' for individuals with such positive, adaptive characteristics and support systems that promote resilience."[6]

But "'toxic stress'" occurs when the person affected "has limited support and . . . may also have brain architecture that reflects effects of adverse early life events that have impaired the development of good impulse control and judgment and adequate self esteem."[7] This was my state of being and is the main focus of my argument here. Because of my accumulated experiences within the past decade, I could not cope normally, which caused adverse effects in my behavior, my overall outlook, and my physiology. Therefore, it is vital that we understand that unrelenting stress and a dominant motivator of fear are not without consequences.

Spirit, soul, and body—they're all connected. Proverbs 14:30 validates this point: "A calm and undisturbed mind and heart are the life and health of the body, but envy, jealousy, and wrath are like rottenness of the bones" (AMPC). What drives envy, jealousy, and wrath? An underlying motivation of fear, which causes a stress response in our physiology.

But what does this have to do with willpower? What does this have to do with the desire and effort to change our lives and move forward, especially after a significant loss or personal defeat?

Everything. Stay with me as I build my case. I believe you will not only be freed from fruitless efforts to change the course of your life, but you'll also learn, like me, to relinquish the self-protective, fear-driven penchant toward survival, control, and independence.

Here's some science to establish my argument: In a state of chronic stress, the sympathetic nervous system remains in drive too long, because the hypothalamic-pituitary-adrenal (HPA) axis in the brain is continuously activated. And like a motor idling too high for an extended period of time, problems then arise within our bodies.[8] In fact, medical research estimates that as much as 95 percent of all illness is related to stress.[9] Moreover, regarding stress and brain function, "researchers believe that when one part of the brain is engaged, the other parts may not have as much energy to handle their own vital tasks."[10] Dr. Kerry Ressler, chief scientific officer at McLean Hospital and psychiatry professor at Harvard Medical School said, "The basic idea is that the brain is shunting its resources because it's in survival mode, not memory mode."[11] This is why stress affects one's memory and overall mood. In this case, the prolonged stress diverts energy from brain regions that manage higher-order tasks—such as the prefrontal cortex, where we think critically and logically, make decisions, and exert willpower—to the more primitive "survival brain," otherwise known as the limbic system.[12] The limbic system is the seat of emotions, beliefs, and traumatic memories, where we store subconscious narratives regarding ourselves, our identities, and the world around us.

It's important to understand the far-reaching effects of unmitigated stress, let alone toxic thinking patterns and traumatic memories, because according to a prominent cell biologist, the neurological processing abilities of the subconscious mind are significantly more powerful than that of the conscious mind (*at least* a million times more powerful).[13] Perhaps the most important factor at play is that about 95 percent of our daily lives is run by our subconscious minds, leaving only 5 percent to our conscious minds.[14] This means that the stress (fear) response to life, including traumatic memories and core beliefs, is far more powerful than any assertion of desire, intention, or willpower in a given situation. In other words, no amount of willpower stands a chance at moving your life from trauma to transformation—to healing what can't be erased.

Again, please understand that the three-step willpower playbook (in which you set your intention, create a plan, and then act on the plan) is not inherently the problem. In fact, articulating what we want to accomplish in life, especially in writing, has countless benefits. But if we're depending on *willpower* to change not only our situations but also *us* from the inside out—particularly when we've lived in an elevated state of stress and survival for any length of time—we're building a house of cards. It's designed to fail from the get-go.

> If we're depending on *willpower* to change not only our situations but also *us* from the inside out–particularly when we've lived in an elevated state of stress and survival for any length of time–we're building a house of cards. It's designed to fail from the get-go.

This is precisely why we don't have what it takes to fix or heal ourselves. While we can position ourselves for healing, we cannot turn the key to systemic life transformation by our own determination, desire, or will. It's why so many of us fail to execute the things we really want to do. And in many cases, we end up doing the things we don't want to do—just like the apostle Paul.

THE WILL WITHOUT THE POWER

In Romans 7, we're presented with a wrestle of sorts: Paul's fight between knowing what is right (and wanting to implement that knowledge) and being unable to follow through with action. In verse 15, Paul said, "I do not understand my own actions. For I do not do what I want, but I do the very thing I hate." In other words, Paul said he had the will but not the power to do what he wanted to do.[15]

And like Paul, though we might have the will, ultimately we lack the power to exact meaningful, transformative change in our lives. Verse 18 in the New Living Translation confirms the same: "I know that nothing good lives in me, that is, in my sinful nature. I want to do what is right, *but I can't.*"

Allow me a quick aside. I believe it is absolutely critical to handle the Word of God studiously, fully apprehending the context of the writing. The scriptural context of Romans 7 is not Paul's ability to set and achieve goals or overcome loss. As a measure of personal integrity, I want to be diligent to not read my own conclusions into the text or make a point that isn't there; instead, I want to teach the text as it is written. *However,* I believe it is fair to zoom out and recognize the through line that Paul presented in the text: Our human personality's *limited ability* to act on what it desires or wills apart from the Holy Spirit's power at work within us. Paul might have had the will, but he lacked the power. And so it is with us.

TRANSFORMATION TAKES TIME

Changing your life from the inside out—transforming your spirit, soul, and body—will never be the result of willpower. None of us can truly fix, heal, or transform ourselves. Our secularized postmodern culture has built the concepts of self-creation and self-healing into a house and wants you to take up residence in it. But because the house lacks a foundation, it will fall. It's just a matter of time.

And even if you have the will, you do not have unlimited power to change your life. None of us do. My black binder was packed with information and a strategy I considered to be a bulletproof playbook for recovery. But what I needed wasn't more desire, effort, or information. Information alone couldn't change my life, and behavior modification wasn't the answer. What I needed was the power of the Holy Spirit to change my *heart*—something only He can do.

Heart transformation is the difference maker, and the lack thereof is the deal-breaker for every situation we face, because heart transformation is systemic; it affects all we do and all we are. Remember what Solomon wrote? "Above all else, guard your heart, for *everything you do* flows from it."[16]

We will spend a lot more time on the issues of the heart in chapters 9 and 10, but for now, allow me to give you a quick primer on heart transformation. When Solomon wrote "guard your heart," he wasn't teaching about us protecting the physical organ in our chests. In Scripture, *heart* refers to the innermost part of a person's being. It encompasses the mind, will, seat of emotions and desires, and center of belief.[17] Therefore, heart *transformation* is an overhaul of your core beliefs, mindsets, and attitudes about yourself, life, and the people around you.

> Heart transformation is the difference maker, and the lack thereof is the deal-breaker for every situation we face.

Paul put it this way in Ephesians 4:23–24: "Be *constantly renewed* in the spirit of your mind [having a fresh mental and spiritual attitude], and *put on the new nature* (the regenerate self) created in God's image, [Godlike] in true righteousness and holiness" (AMPC). To thrive in life, the transformed heart doesn't depend on the external circumstances changing. Nor does it ignore the sometimes-devastating reality of life. Instead, it acknowledges a greater reality amid our pain and disorientation. This is precisely why our transformed hearts affect not only what we do or how we do it but also who we are and why we do what we do.

Perhaps for the first time in a long while, you're beginning to realize that the change you've been attempting to manufacture in your life requires an entirely different approach—one that is beyond the scope of your own insight, understanding, performance, strength, and ability. For this reason, you must understand that information alone will not incite dynamic, meaningful life change. Good information without consistent application over time, *by the power of the Holy Spirit,* will never produce transformation. And as I said earlier, the self-creation, self-healing narrative is bound to implode eventually, because it is like a house without a solid foundation. Its walls have been built on the lies that say you are the architect of your own destiny, that you can manifest whatever life you desire, that this work of transformation is all on you, and that you must self-protect and self-promote because the disappointment of your past "proves" that God is apparently incapable and unwilling to keep you safe.

Having said this, I know there's a good chance that after what you've endured, you're just exhausted and want help—*any* semblance of help. I completely understand. So, even if you feel overwhelmed about how (or where) to begin to chart your roadmap to wholeness and even if you're rather timid about trusting again, by faith I believe the seed has been planted. The truth is that the Lord has never been absent from your life, even if your perception of His presence told you the opposite.

As has always been the case, unlimited power is available for God's purposes to be accomplished in your life. In Philippians 2:13, Paul wrote, "It is *God* who works in you, *both to will and to work* for his good pleasure." Look at the Amplified Bible Classic Edition's translation of this verse: "[Not in your own strength] for it is God Who is all the while effectually at work in you [energizing and creating in you the power and desire], both to will and to work for His good pleasure and satisfaction and delight." And there it is. *God* gives us the *will* and the *power* for life. Without question, transformation is indeed the better path and wholeness is the better destination. Therefore, if heart transformation by the renewing of the mind beats willpower-driven self-help and if transformation by God's Spirit is the pathway to experience systemic life change, what's required of us? The answer, I believe, is TIME:

T = Total surrender. A transformed life is a surrendered life—a humble, teachable life that recognizes it cannot change or heal itself. And a humble, teachable life is a *planted* life. Indeed, I believe this soul posture is the foundation of healing and transformation. In teaching His disciples in John 15:1–5, Jesus said,

> I am the true vine, and my Father is the vinedresser. Every branch in me that does not bear fruit he takes away, and every branch that does bear fruit he prunes, that it may bear more fruit. Already you are clean because of the word that I have spoken to you. Abide in me, and I in you. As the branch cannot bear fruit by itself, unless it abides in the vine, neither can you, unless you abide in me. I am the vine; you are the branches. Whoever abides in me and I in him, he it is that bears much fruit, for apart from me you can do nothing.

Craig Keener, a respected biblical scholar, wrote about this passage, saying, "The most basic point of the imagery is the obvious dependence of branches on the vine for their continued life." Also of distinct relevance to our context, he noted that "both Jewish and Greek sources" applied the word *prunes* (meaning "cleanses") "to inward purification of the heart."[18] This is why I believe the extent to which the Lord can entrust us with influence, oversight, resources, and responsibilities is predicated on the extent to which we allow Him access to confront, correct, teach, heal, and love us from the inside out. This is total surrender, a posture of the heart that cries, "Lord, have Your way in me!" How does this occur practically? We must prioritize the time we spend in the Scriptures, prayer, personal worship and communion with Him, and fellowship with other believers—specifically those who will help us grow and sharpen us like "iron sharpens iron."[19]

I = Intentional pursuit. Jesus said, "Where your treasure is, there your heart will be also."[20] The actual priorities of our hearts and lives are not hard to spot. Whatever we value most will occupy the greatest real estate in our schedules, reflecting those priorities. How desperate are we for change? How steadfast will we be in pursuing Him to receive freedom and healing for our broken hearts? As Psalm 34:18 says, "The LORD is near to the brokenhearted and saves the crushed in spirit." Make time for Him. Pursue Him. And don't stop. Sometimes, the most honest prayer is one word: "Help!"

M = Mature mindset. In Romans 8:13–17, Paul wrote,

> If you live according to the flesh you will die, but if by the Spirit you put to death the deeds of the body, you will live. For all who are led by the Spirit of God are sons of God. For you did not receive the spirit of slavery to fall back into fear, but you have received the Spirit of adoption as sons, by whom we cry, "Abba! Father!" The Spirit himself bears witness with our spirit that we are children of God, and if children, then heirs—heirs of God and fellow heirs with Christ, provided we suffer with him in order that we may also be glorified with him.[21]

Moreover, 1 Corinthians 14:20 says, "Brothers, do not be children in your thinking. Be infants in evil, but *in your thinking be mature.*" The goal of our Christian experience is maturity, which is the distinction of the "sons of God." And these "sons," men and women led by the Spirit, pursue a mature mindset that empowers them to commit to the daily process of transformation with consistency and character.

E = Eternal motivation. When painful, unrelenting circumstances obstruct our paths, it's easy to miss the forest for the trees. In other words, we miss the long-range perspective we can have as a result of our position in Christ and His eternal purpose for His kingdom. In Romans 8:18, Paul wrote, "I consider that the sufferings of this present time are not worth comparing with the glory that is to be revealed to us." That's why I believe our stewardship of this short life counts for the next life. James wrote, "You do not know what tomorrow will bring. What is your life? For you are a mist that appears for a little time and then vanishes."[22] God's eternal purpose, etched in history from the foundation of the earth, will be accomplished. And we are part of His eternal purpose! How exciting is that? This begs the question, What are you doing with *today*? Here's Jesus from Matthew 6:27–34 for a little reminder:

> Which of you by being anxious can add a single hour to his span of life? And why are you anxious about clothing? Consider the lilies of the field, how they grow: they neither toil nor spin, yet I tell you, even Solomon in all his glory was not arrayed like one of these. But if God so clothes the grass of the field, which today is alive and tomorrow is thrown into the oven, will he not much more clothe you, O you of little faith? Therefore *do not be anxious,* saying, "What shall we eat?" or "What shall we drink?" or "What shall we wear?" For the Gentiles seek after all these things, and your heavenly Father knows that you need them all. But seek first the kingdom of God and his righteousness, and all these things will be added to you. Therefore *do not be anxious about tomorrow,* for tomorrow will be anxious for itself. Sufficient for the day is its own trouble.

TIME, my friend, will calibrate the affections of your heart to Jesus in such a way that will rouse transformation from the inside out, because a transformed life is an effective, overcoming life.

Sadly, however, too many of us stay stuck, repeating patterns that don't catalyze systemic change, because we've used self-creation and self-healing as a substitute for true Holy Spirit–empowered formation and transformation according to the way and practice of Jesus. But the truth is that you do not have to self-protect, self-promote, and take care of yourself any longer. You don't have to perform your way to wholeness. Your past disappointments may seem to make a plausible case that God is incapable of keeping you safe—or worse, unwilling to do so. Yet please trust me when I implore you (from personal experience) to relinquish your penchant toward an independent spirit, even when it doesn't make sense to your rational mind. There is a better option.

LIVING BEYOND OURSELVES

Paul's magnum opus in Romans exemplifies my point. It starts in 11:36: "From him and through him and to him are all things. To him be glory forever. Amen." And the very next two verses, verses 1 and 2 of chapter 12, implore us to "present your bodies as a living sacrifice, holy and acceptable to God, which is your spiritual worship. *Do not be conformed* to this world, *but be transformed* by the renewal of your mind, that by testing you may discern what is the will of God, what is good and acceptable and perfect."

The Message paraphrases this passage brilliantly:

Here's what I want you to do, God helping you: Take your everyday, ordinary life—your sleeping, eating, going-to-work, and walking-around life—and place it before God as an offering. Embracing what God does for you is the best thing you can do for him. Don't become so well-adjusted to your culture that you fit into it *without even thinking.* Instead, *fix your attention on God.* You'll be changed from the inside out. Readily recognize what he wants from you, and quickly respond to it. Unlike the culture around you, always dragging you down to its level of immaturity, God brings the best out of you, develops well-formed maturity in you.

What is the world's pattern of thinking? *Trust yourself. Follow your heart. Live your truth. Look inside yourself to find the truth of who you are.* But, my friend, it's a trap. When your locus of authority and guidance is yourself, you are bound for shipwreck.

At the end of the day, the step toward freedom and wholeness is your choice. So, will you come out of hiding? Will you surrender your penchant toward independence? Will you be honest about your trust issues? Will you ask for help? Will you receive fresh wisdom from the One "who gives generously to all without reproach"?[23] Who told you that your freedom and healing were all up to you anyway? Because they aren't.

Having said that, our perpetual sense of defeat also has a more insidious cause. I know it all too well because I was on the verge of utter collapse. It pulses from deep within us. And I believe it is the linchpin reason why many of us stay stuck for far too long. I'm speaking of the wounded, broken spirit.

PERSONALIZE IT

THE POINT

We don't have what it takes to fix or heal ourselves. While we can position ourselves for healing, we cannot turn the key to systemic life transformation by our own determination, desire, or will.

THE PROMPT

Ask the Holy Spirit to show you areas in which you're depending on your own insight, understanding, or ability for change, growth, and healing—areas that are perhaps lacking total surrender, intentional pursuit, a mature mindset, and an eternal motivation. Your trust *in* the Lord is proportional to your surrender *to* Him. Be ready to listen thoroughly and respond (with action) to what He shows you.

THE POSTURE

Whatever we value most will occupy the greatest real estate in our schedules, reflecting the priorities of our hearts. Do you desire sustainable growth in your life? Then make practical choices that reflect your desire. Small changes applied daily add up over time, so start today. Moreover, in this process, allow the Lord's correction to come where shortsightedness or immaturity abounds. This isn't easy. Confrontation is rarely fun, but your willingness to address the issues He reveals to you will yield greater effectiveness in your life.

THE PRAYER

Lord, You have given me the ability and responsibility to steward my life. And while I can exercise that stewardship by learning, growing, and developing each day, I cannot turn the key to transformation. So today, I ask You to teach me how to surrender my self-dependency and instead trust in and lean on Your strength. I ask for the will and the power to do what You have called me to do for Your good pleasure. Amen.

THREE

_____

THE BROKEN SPIRIT

A healthy spirit conquers adversity,
but what can you do when the spirit is crushed?

—PROVERBS 18:14, MSG

I want to rewind the tape to a time before my encounter with the Lord in October 2014 when He asked me the pivotal question, "What do you want Me to do for you?" Most mornings for about seven months, between September 2013 and April 2014, tears welled up in my eyes even before I was fully awake. As I dragged myself out from my covers, dread headlined each new day before my feet hit the floor. Though my legs hung off the side of my bed, it was as if the rest of my body, with an almost calculated rebellion, fought the burgeoning dawn light that pierced through my window blinds. With pain and numbness shooting through my limbs, all I wanted to do was collapse back onto my pillow.

Ten or fifteen minutes would pass before I could break myself from the emotional weight draped across my back and wrapped around my chest. It wasn't a comforting embrace by any stretch. Instead, it was like a heavy tapestry knit by depression, chronic fatigue, and trauma, custom designed and fitted for me, express shipped from the nightmare that was my everyday life. And despite a full night's sleep, I met each morning with physical pain and soul-deep exhaustion. Night sweats were a regular occurrence, too, due to my body's weaning from the heavy corticosteroids prescribed after my MS diagnosis. That experience scared me all by itself because when I was a little boy, night sweats were one of my mom's earliest symptoms of cancer.

Needless to say, panic and irrational fear piled on my soul in an unremitting manner. As I previously mentioned, every day during my lunch break, I'd set my alarm for twenty-five minutes and try to take a nap, though I'd end up bursting into tears and sobbing for most of that time. I was barely existing. Hours turned into days, and days into weeks. Seasons passed. I created a very safe but stuck life because it's all I knew to do. The numbness was pervasive and didn't take a day off. Most days before work, I'd lie on my bedroom floor and cry, feeling so tired and so alone. Candidly, I ended most nights in the same position. But even ten hours of sleep at night didn't alleviate the spirit-deep brokenness I felt.

One of the scariest nights of this time occurred on a Saturday during one of Michigan's dark winter months. I was home alone and decided to go to bed early, because somehow I felt safer there with my eyes closed. It was like I didn't have to see the world for what it really was or accidentally catch a glimpse of my leaden countenance in the mirror. But as I buried my head under the covers, I began to hear my mom screaming in pain. "Don't leave me!" she cried. Granted, Mom had been gone for more than a year, but the screams heard only inside my mind sent chills down my spine. It felt as real as ever.

I pulled the covers tighter to my body as sweat began to drench my undershirt and my bedsheets. Shaking violently and lying in the fetal position, I felt trapped. I wanted this nightmare to end, but those silent screams would not relent. Somehow after fifteen or twenty minutes, I had the intuition to call two of my best friends. Struggling to put words together, I tried to describe what was happening until one of them interrupted me midstream and told me to get in the car and drive over. I did exactly that, and for the next three hours or so, I sat at their kitchen island, mostly silent, heavy tears dripping into the cup of hot tea they fixed for me.

We didn't say much that night, but we didn't need to. What I needed more than anything (and what I received) was their loving presence. Those two had been a rock in my life for years. Not just friends, they had become family. I trusted them with my life, and they regularly came through in a way that probably saved it more than once.

The inescapable, unswerving sense of lifelessness and defeat was like nothing I had ever experienced. It was deeper than grief. With grief, I could separate my feelings from my identity. But this? This became a part of me. I was it; it was me. And *it* was a broken spirit that was suffocating my hope and atrophying my livelihood in a slow, devastating manner.

Frankly, not enough people talk about a wounded, broken spirit—not even in the church. But it's a silent killer, as lethal today as it has been for thousands of years. Enter the children of Israel.

LEAVING EGYPT WITHOUT EGYPT LEAVING YOU

After their long period of captivity in Egypt, the children of Israel were led to exodus by Moses, which not only ended their oppression by Pharoah and the Egyptians but also inaugurated the fulfillment of the Lord's covenant with Abraham, made generations prior, when He instructed, "Go from your country and your kindred and your father's house to the land that I will show you. And I will make of you a great nation, and I will bless you and make your name great, so that you will be a blessing."[1]

Tragically, however, the Israelites' exodus proved that even though they got out of Egypt, "Egypt" never got out of them. Let's pick up the story in Exodus 14:10–12, just prior to their crossing the Red Sea:

> When Pharaoh drew near, the people of Israel lifted up their eyes, and behold, the Egyptians were marching after them, *and they feared greatly*. And the people of Israel cried out to the LORD. They said to Moses, "Is it because there are no

graves in Egypt that you have taken us away to die in the wilderness? What have you done to us in bringing us out of Egypt? Is not this what we said to you in Egypt: 'Leave us alone that we may serve the Egyptians'? For *it would have been better for us to serve the Egyptians than to die in the wilderness.*"

"Leave us alone," they demanded. How quickly they forgot their former condition and thus argued that it would be better to live in slavery than to die in freedom. And even though Moses told them to "fear not, stand firm, and see the salvation of the LORD,"[2] clearly fear had penetrated their hearts, and cynicism about the Lord's goodness was leading their minds—perhaps from the trauma and bitterness of spending years in hard service and ruthless work as the Egyptian rulers' slaves.[3]

The sequence of events that followed resulted in the miraculous parting of the Red Sea, after which the children of Israel sang a song of victory to the Lord. And though the hand of the Lord worked many more miracles in the people's presence, their momentary satisfaction inevitably gave way to murmuring, grumbling, and eventually rebellion. In Numbers 13, the Lord told Moses to send men into Canaan to spy out the Promised Land. Upon their return, the spies told Moses and Aaron, "We came to the land to which you sent us. It flows with milk and honey, and this is its fruit. However, the people who dwell in the land are strong, and the cities are fortified and very large. And besides, we saw the descendants of Anak there."[4]

The people's response to this report must have incited an uproar, because moments later, Caleb—one of the spies giving the report—"quieted the people before Moses and said, 'Let us go up at once and occupy it, for we are well able to overcome it.' "[5]

Look at the two different responses to the spies' account: The people, obviously overwhelmed by a spirit of fear, cried out in panic. But Caleb, despite the true description of Canaan's inhabitants, remained steadfast, trusting that regardless of the obstacles before them, the Lord would be faithful to lead and strengthen them to overcome. What was the difference between Caleb and the people? *The state of their spirits.* Let's continue.

Sadly, the other spies continued to bring a fearful report to the people, saying, "The land, through which we have gone to spy it out, is a land that devours its inhabitants, and all the people that we saw in it are of great height. And there we saw the Nephilim (the sons of Anak, who come from the Nephilim), and *we seemed to ourselves like grasshoppers, and so we seemed to them.*"[6]

Despite the Lord's promise to the people, their perspective about their position determined the posture by which they would live and lead. And what followed was nothing short of chaotic rebellion. Aroused by fear and anger, they said to Moses and Aaron:

> "Would that we had died in the land of Egypt! Or would that we had died in this wilderness! Why is the LORD bringing us into this land, to fall by the sword? Our wives and our little ones will become a prey. Would it not be better for us to go back to Egypt?" And they said to one another, "Let us choose a leader and go back to Egypt."[7]

Did they not see the promise of the Lord to be with them in their conquest? Or could they not see it because of the condition of their hearts? As Moses and Aaron fell on their faces before the people, Joshua and Caleb, full of passion and determined to see the promise of the Lord, urged:

> The land, which we passed through to spy it out, is an exceedingly good land. If the LORD delights in us, he will bring us into this land and give it to us, a land that flows with milk and honey. *Only do not rebel against the LORD. And do not fear the people of the land,* for they are bread for us. Their protection is removed from them, and the LORD is with us; do not fear them.[8]

The Lord then responded to Moses: "How long will this people despise me? And how long will they not believe in me, in spite of all the signs that I have done among them? I will strike them with the pestilence and disinherit them, and I will make of you a nation greater and mightier than they."[9]

He'd had enough. Perhaps He would wipe out the people and start afresh. Moses, however, standing as the friend of God he was,[10] interceded before the Lord on the people's behalf:

> If you kill this people as one man, then the nations who have heard your fame will say, "It is because the LORD was not able to bring this people into the land that he swore to give to them that he has killed them in the wilderness." And now, please let the power of the Lord be great as you have promised, saying, "The LORD is slow to anger and abounding in steadfast love, forgiving iniquity and transgression, but he will by no means clear the guilty, visiting the iniquity of the fathers on the children, to the third and the fourth generation." Please pardon the iniquity of this people, according to the greatness of your steadfast love, just as you have forgiven this people, from Egypt until now.[11]

Once again, the Lord would indeed forgive the people, but because of their insistent rebellion, He declared that this generation of people would not live to see the Promised Land[12]—that is, except for Joshua and Caleb. About Caleb, the Lord said, "My servant Caleb, *because he has a different spirit* and has followed me fully, I will bring into the land into which he went, and his descendants shall possess it."[13]

Two million people had been delivered from slavery, yet "slavery" (embodied by self-protection, cynicism, and an independent, rebellious spirit) remained in them. Bitterness, fear, distrust, and distress dominated the climate of their souls. It was why they lived for so long under the influence of a broken spirit[14]—and why you and I, today, are susceptible to the same condition.

The Wind in the Sail

The Hebrew word for "spirit" in this context is *ruach,* which is often translated as "breath" or "wind."[15] But when the Bible speaks of our human spirit, especially in the book of Proverbs, *ruach* refers to our inner drive for life, our courage and vigor, and the animation of our being. Think about it this way: If your body were a boat and your soul were a sail that steered the boat's direction, your spirit would be the wind and force that give life and motion to the sail. When our spirits are broken—when the wind in our sails is absent, perhaps because of physical, mental, or emotional unhealth; a moral failure; a loved one's death; or a relationship's collapse—our passion, drive, and desire for life are gone too.

In this experience, we're not talking merely about a difficult season either. We're talking about an unrelenting, all-encompassing sense of utter defeat and despair. And even if a person's life looks put together from the outside, it will not flourish long-term under the influence of a broken, wounded spirit. Proverbs 18:14 exemplifies this point brilliantly: "The human spirit can endure in sickness, but a *crushed spirit* who can bear?" (NIV). In other words, in the presence of a healthy spirit, a sick, broken body can be made well. But under the weight of a broken spirit, not even a healthy body will flourish long-term. Again, because your spirit, soul, and body are all connected, a broken spirit will affect you in a systemic manner.

Perhaps more than any other book of the Bible, Proverbs speaks about the origin and expression of a broken spirit. Here are a few key examples:

A gentle tongue is a tree of life,
  but perverseness in it breaks the spirit. (15:4)

A glad heart makes a cheerful face,
  but by sorrow of heart the spirit is crushed. (15:13)

A joyful heart is good medicine,
    but a crushed spirit dries up the bones. (17:22)

A man's spirit will endure sickness,
    but a crushed spirit who can bear? (18:14)

THE CYCLE OF PAIN

As you can see, the conversation around the broken spirit is a complex issue that affects us physically, emotionally, and even relationally. But what leads to the moment when the spirit is broken? Is there a buildup of unmitigated pain and loss before that happens? And what can we learn from human behavior, Scripture, and neuroscience about how to predict and prevent a state of being (a new identity) forged by fear, shame, blame, victimhood, and despair?

I want to take you inside the following diagram of the cycle of pain, which I created and have been using for about six years. It paints a picture of the ideal culture (think of a greenhouse) in which a broken spirit thrives and the reasons it can so insidiously become a person's normal state of being, even though it's anything but normal. Not only was this my personal experience, but many of my coaching clients have also experienced it. Have a look:

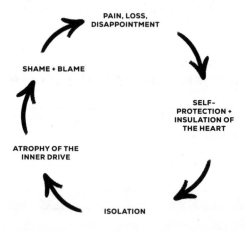

Here's how the cycle of pain plays out: All of us will experience a measure of pain, loss, disappointment, hurt, or betrayal in life. It's an issue not of "if," but of "when"—you know this as well as I do. For me, the accumulation of painful circumstances and an unrelenting climate of fear that ruled my heart over the course of two decades culminated with my mom's death and my multiple sclerosis diagnosis nine months later. For the children of Israel, the breaking point was arguably the moment described in Exodus 1 in which the Egyptians "set taskmasters over them to afflict them with heavy burdens. . . . *So they ruthlessly made the people of Israel work as slaves and made their lives bitter* with hard service, in mortar and brick, and in all kinds of work in the field. In all their work they ruthlessly made them work as slaves."[16]

What was it for you? A vicious divorce? The death of a loved one? The betrayal by a significant other? Whether it happened five years or five minutes ago, pain is pain, and it must be acknowledged as such. I don't want to ignore the physiological responses from our sympathetic nervous system in stressful, alarming moments of life like these, but in this context, I'm going to focus less on science and more on what happens within our hearts from a spiritual perspective. In doing so, I hope you'll observe the ideal climate in which a broken spirit thrives (and stays broken) and learn how to address it now and in the future. After all, it's been said, "As hard as the initial trauma is, it's the aftermath that destroys people."[17] And thus the exploration of this cycle of pain is an attempt to identify and mitigate these core issues that put a stranglehold on our drive for life.

If phase one is the inciting moment of pain or loss, phase two involves protecting ourselves and insulating our hearts in an effort to make sure we don't experience that same pain again. I coped with my pain by shrinking my options and my life's boundary lines. I created as much predictability in my routine as possible, because history had proven that surprises were rarely good. A small life, I contended, was a *safe* life. But what was happening to my heart in the process? A callus of skepticism turned cynicism began to form. And in time, had I not sought help, I think it would have turned into unbelief.

Think about your own life. After a painful experience such as, say, a relationship breakup, what's a common response? Do you determine that you'll never ever let this happen again? And if so, how do you set up parameters of protection over your heart? Does your level of trust go down while your level of self-reliance goes up? And just to be clear, I'm not at all implying that we shouldn't learn from dysfunctional behavior patterns in a relationship, become wiser, enact change, establish new and healthy boundaries, and so forth. Boundaries in every relationship are good and necessary. Rather, I'm talking about a *heart posture* motivated by fear, doubt, cynicism, and self-reliance, not interdependence, humility, growth, and learning.

Let's go back to the children of Israel. Regarding their "phase two" experience, Scripture says, "I was provoked with that generation, and said, 'They always go astray in their heart; they have not known my ways.' As I swore in my wrath, 'They shall not enter my rest.'"[18] Because of the unmitigated systemic fear and pain instigated by their slavery in Egypt, they developed distrust for both Moses and God in the wilderness, *even though they never once lacked provision or protection.* This distrust led to rebellion, resulting in the inability for that generation of Israelites to enter the Promised Land. And as this scripture from Hebrews reveals, the ticking time bomb was not in their words or actions but in their hearts. Their *perspective* about their *position* in life determined the *posture* by which they lived their lives. It bears repeating: Even though they were taken out of Egypt, "Egypt" never left them. And even though you might be years past a devastating loss, betrayal, diagnosis, or disappointment, that loss—whatever it is—might still be informing how you engage with life and the Lord Himself on a daily basis.

Phase three of the cycle of pain arrives in our hearts more insidiously than phase two, because it's an outgrowth of self-protection over time. I'm speaking of isolation. It's one thing to make boundary-based decisions about the extent to which people have access to your life. And that's wise. But isolating yourself from *all* relationships eliminates the good, healthy, life-giving ones too—including the Lord. And that's not only unwise; it's deadly. The scariest part about isolation is that we rarely recognize that it's happening. It's like the slow drift of a raft at sea. Small but steady movements away from the shore eventually leave the raft stranded and alone in the wide-open water. Worse, when we isolate ourselves, we cut off our connection to the Vine Himself. Remember what Jesus told His disciples in John 15?

> I am the true vine, and my Father is the vinedresser. Every branch in me that does not bear fruit he takes away, and every branch that does bear fruit he prunes, that it may bear more fruit. Already you are clean because of the word that I have spoken to you. Abide in me, and I in you. As the branch cannot bear fruit by itself, unless it abides in the vine, neither can you, unless you abide in me. I am the vine; you are the branches. Whoever abides in me and I in him, he it is that bears much fruit, for apart from me you can do nothing. If anyone does not abide in me he is thrown away like a branch and withers; and the branches are gathered, thrown into the fire, and burned. If you abide in me, and my words abide in you, ask whatever you wish, and it will be done for you.[19]

Staying connected to the Vine is critical because what's at stake is more than our peace—it's our very reason to live.

We were designed for an ongoing transformative process whose goal is union with God. And while nothing can separate us from the love of God,[20] we, through an act of our free will, can separate ourselves from Him. Said another way, "God is always present, but we are not always present to God."[21] And the lethal nature of separateness cannot be overstated. In separating ourselves, not only are we severed from our source of life and truth, who is Christ, but we also become vulnerable to receiving and believing lies that drive us deeper into a self-focused, self-created, self-protective, cynical life of bitterness and despair. Little by little, seeds of doubt are sowed into our minds. *You can't trust anyone. Where is your God now? If He loved you, would He have let this happen . . . again? He just failed you like everyone else. Trust only yourself. Keep your heart at a distance from people. It's safer.* And slowly but surely, we believe them. Proverbs 18:1 validates this idea: "Whoever isolates himself seeks his own desire; he breaks out against all sound judgment." Wisdom and truth are absent where isolation abounds, because where isolation abounds, deception thrives. Safety is indeed found in a multitude of healthy, wise counselors.[22]

Let's take a quick moment to review the trajectory of this cycle as presented thus far. Phase one is the initial moment of wounding. Because this is bound to happen many times throughout life, my prayer for you going forward, having immersed yourself in learning how this cycle of pain works, is that you will seek help and counsel immediately, before a callus of self-protection begins to take shape over your heart in phase two. When self-protection becomes one's default state in life, it isn't long before isolation sets in, which is phase three.

After isolating and removing ourselves from our source of life, like a branch cut off from the Vine, we step into phase four, which is most often characterized by defeat and despair—a perpetual state of ennui. Most certainly, it's the suffocation and atrophy of our hope and expectation for life. At the height of his pain and grief, Job said in despair, "My spirit is broken; my days are extinct; the graveyard is ready for me."[23] The Hebrew word for "broken" here is *châbal* (pronounced *khaw-bal'*), which, according to *Strong's Concordance,* means "to wind tightly (as a rope)" or "to bind."[24] Imagine a rope tied around your arm tightly enough to cut off the circulation of blood. What would happen eventually? Obviously, the limb would atrophy. In the same way, stifling our life source suffocates and atrophies our human spirits. Danish theologian Søren Kierkegaard called this despair "the sickness unto death."[25]

At this point, a common recourse is to turn to shame and blame. Shame internalizes the pain and adopts it as part of our identity. No longer is the ordeal or loss an experience; it is an inseparable part of who we are. Repudiating the truth that we are "fearfully and wonderfully made,"[26] shame crowns us with the false identity of "uniquely and fatally flawed without remedy." And in unison, blame declares to the Lord and to those we have looked to for safety and security, "If you would have loved me, this wouldn't have happened!"

Remember what Adam told God after he sinned in the garden? "The woman whom you gave to be with me, she gave me fruit of the tree, and I ate."[27] Of course, the children of Israel were no different when they complained to Moses, "What have you done to us in bringing us out of Egypt? Is not this what we said to you in Egypt: 'Leave us alone that we may serve the Egyptians'? For it would have been better for us to serve the Egyptians than to die in the wilderness."[28]

Worse, because of the broken spirit, the cycle of pain has the potential to repeat indefinitely. Having turned to shame and blame, we feel more pain and loss, causing us to insulate our hearts and hunker down in self-protection all the more, which leads to greater depths of isolation, which "ties the rope" even tighter, which results in an even more caustic expression of shame and blame in our daily lives. As we've already said, this level of distress is most certain to wreak havoc on our bodies.

Bessel van der Kolk, in writing about the anatomy of survival in *The Body Keeps the Score,* said, "Being traumatized means continuing to organize your life as if the trauma were still going on—unchanged and immutable—as every new encounter or event is contained by the past."[29] He continued,

> After trauma the world is experienced with a different nervous system. The survivor's energy now becomes focused on suppressing inner chaos, at the expense of spontaneous involvement in their life. These attempts to maintain control over unbearable physiological reactions can result in a whole range of physical symptoms, including fibromyalgia, chronic fatigue, and other autoimmune diseases. This explains why

it is critical for trauma treatment to engage the entire organism, body, mind, and brain.[30]

Again, let's frame this wisdom up against Scripture. Proverbs 14:30 says, "A calm and undisturbed mind and heart are the life and health of the body, but envy, jealousy, and wrath are like rottenness of the bones" (AMPC). Moreover, the apostle John wrote, "Beloved, I pray that all may go well with you and that you may be in good health, as it goes well with your soul."[31] See? It's all connected.

This is precisely why the aim of this book is to steer our priorities toward transformation, not simply recovery, because transformation and restoration are values of the kingdom. The prophet Joel said, "I will restore or replace for you the years that the locust has eaten."[32] It's one thing to recover that which was lost. But it's entirely more transformative and significant to experience restoration by the hand of the Lord. He doesn't simply refurbish. He *replaces* for the glory of His great name.

Therefore, the priority of dealing with the inner life cannot be overstated. This is why in chapter 2 I proposed that heart transformation beats willpower-driven self-help (behavior modification) every time. As Solomon's words will indeed be a cornerstone of this entire book, I remind you that we are to "keep and guard" our hearts above all else, for everything we do and are emanates from that place.[33]

> Nothing is more important than maintaining your inner life.

Nothing is more important than maintaining your inner life. Much of the self-help industry and popular psychology approaches this subject one-dimensionally.[34] Too often, we hit behavior modification but miss heart transformation that will change our lives from the inside out. Each of us is more than a body. We are more than our emotions and certainly more than our desires or thoughts. All of those things are vital to address.

But most importantly, we are complex beings who were intricately woven together fearfully and wonderfully in our mothers' wombs by the hand and design of almighty God. And this is why most self-help solutions are short-lived and incomplete. They lack nuance and discernment regarding the complexity of the inner life and its effects on every other domain of living.[35] Most of all, I believe it is critical to understand that because the root issue is spiritual, the necessary healing is spiritual in nature as well. Thus, as we continue to pursue this dynamic work of healing and trans-formation of the inner life, we must explore the tenets of shame, for I believe shame is a dominant player that sustains the life of our broken spirits.

PERSONALIZE IT

THE POINT

Healing a broken, crushed spirit is a linchpin to transformation. Under the influence of a broken spirit, a person experiences an unrelenting and all-encompassing sense of utter defeat and despair. In other words, their inner drive for life is gone.

THE PROMPT

In which area(s) of your life do bitterness, fear, distrust, and distress regularly dominate the climate of your soul? How about self-protection, unbelief, unforgiveness, or cynicism? Are your drive and desire for life absent? And are you isolating yourself not only from your community of believers but also from the Lord Himself?

THE POSTURE

If you are stuck in the cycle of pain, which is perpetuated by shame and blame, there is an invitation to change, to surrender your pain to the Lord, and to move toward the liberating truth of Christ. How? Through honest vulnerability, personal responsibility, and a commitment to allow the ongoing work of the Holy Spirit in your life. So, will you? Don't hesitate another day.

THE PRAYER

Lord, I know that nothing is more important than maintaining my inner life. Today, Lord—maybe for the first time—I surrender my broken spirit to You. And that means I give You every disappointment, loss, and betrayal. I surrender self-protection and repent of my reflex to turn to shame and blame instead of You as a solution to my pain. I willingly come out of hiding and am ready to move forward. I ask You to breathe new life in me. Restore my drive and passion for life once again. Amen.

PART II

THE BUILDING

FOUR

WHEN SHAME ARRIVES

*To be shame-bound means that whenever you feel any
feeling, need or drive, you immediately feel ashamed.
The dynamic core of your human life is grounded in your
feelings, needs and drives. When these are bound by
shame, you are shamed to the core.*

—JOHN BRADSHAW, *Healing the Shame That Binds You*

He sat across the table from me at the restaurant and threw a contemptuous assault straight at my heart: "What . . . are you like a *whore* or something?" I've never been accused of anything, let alone had my character called into question, but the insecure, fear-driven anger that spewed from his mouth in those eight words drove a dagger into my spirit. For forty-five minutes, the berating continued. *What have I actually done wrong?* Cold droplets of perspiration beaded across my brow as I tried to recover coherence following the execution of my self-worth by someone I trusted and respected.

I guess it's true that the size of the weapon doesn't determine its lethal power. It felt like an ice-cold arrow had been shot straight into my heart, and my chest pounded with anxiety and intense pressure as my arms and legs went limp and numb. As I peeled myself off the seat, a burst of nausea and dizziness overwhelmed me. I labored to walk to my car, where I called a mentor and counselor named Dave (whom you'll learn more about in chapter 6). He could help me process what had just transpired.

"Hey, Chris," Dave answered.

Silence. I couldn't speak.

"*Chris?*" he pressed.

I squeaked out four words, "*I. Can. Barely. Breathe.*"

Ten minutes or so later, I was able to put a sentence together to recall the experience to him. Fuming, he talked me off the ledge and then prayed for me. While I felt more stable within a few hours after the incident, my thoughts continued to race unrestrained, for the weapon that had been formed against me was indeed prospering—or at least felt like it was. The tongue that had risen up against me I wanted to refute, but doing so was difficult after having been ambushed and pummeled by such an unsubstantiated berating.

For years, I had heard it said that those closest to you can wound you the deepest, and that day, I found out it was true. I've never been a person to shirk responsibility, so even as a child, I eagerly sought to face circumstantial guilt and own up to my mistakes. If I made a mistake or hurt someone, I wanted to remedy my error as quickly as possible and pursue reconciliation. I hated feeling tension and guilt. But this? *This* experience was different, though familiar.

Pulling back the curtain of my heart, I realize that I've struggled with shame for as long as I can remember. Insidiously, it knit together the belief that despite my best intentions and efforts, the lowest common denominator in any situation was always and forever *me*. And though it's difficult to admit, the core wounded belief was that I was uniquely and inescapably flawed—not for what I had or hadn't done but simply for who I was.

Sadly, even through my young adult years, my attempts to address this root of shame were rarely aimed at healing. It's not that I didn't *want* to heal; rather, I didn't know how to heal or where to start. The voice of shame was all too familiar. In fact, I allowed it to become the loudest in my life. My interaction with this familiar yet devious shame narrative was akin to futile, exhausting attempts at negotiation with a narcissist or emotionally abusive person. Hence, the tornadic shame spiral I was swept into at that restaurant took me back to one of my earliest memories of shame, which I still remember like it was yesterday, even though it occurred when I was only seven or eight years old.

SHAME AS OLD AS ME

I was walking down a neighborhood sidewalk with a trusted adult and didn't see a piece of fruit that had fallen underfoot. As I stepped on it, juice squirted up my leg and onto my clean shorts. I honestly didn't see the fruit. It was an accident, and I was just a little boy. Immediately, she began to scream at me, "How could you be so blind? You have nothing else to wear! You're useless! As smart as you are, why are you so stupid sometimes? This is your fault, and you're going to have to fix this yourself!"

So, I did. And for the next several years, I tried to fix everything else myself too. What ensued throughout my teenage and young adult years was a life motivated by self-protection, insecurity, and perfectionism. I couldn't make a mistake, because if I did, my broken belief system validated that *I* was a mistake.

My first couple of years at an all-boys parochial high school renowned for its athletic tradition were really hard. Not possessing significant height or an athletic frame completely repudiated my ability to fit in with my peers, and I suffered a substantial amount of bullying. No honor roll or 4.0 grade point average could mend the broken place in my soul. My academic stature could never compensate for my insufficient physical stature. And the writing on the wall seemed to confirm once again that the problem wasn't my circumstances; it was *me*. Just to run a thread through the chronology, keep in mind this was only a couple of years after my mom's cancer diagnosis.

All throughout that time, my young mind was writing a story, and I was the main character. In my immaturity, I didn't know how to separate my identity and inherent value from the adversity around me, so I reasoned that I must have played a part in causing it. *If there wasn't something fundamentally flawed with me,* I argued, *these bad things wouldn't be happening.* This was the story I was telling myself, and it was the only way I could make sense of the pain I was experiencing and keep myself as safe as possible each day. Can you relate?

THE STORIES WE TELL OURSELVES

We human beings are wired for story, and we all write them inside the recesses of our minds. Our brains are hardwired to string memories together in narrative form to construct meaning from our life experiences. The stories we tell ourselves form our expectations and hope—our outlook on life. They tell us how to orient ourselves in relation to others. And the reason we tell ourselves stories within our neurobiology is primitive: It's for survival.

Yet there is a personal story that you and I and everyone else share: our story of shame. It started in the garden and continues today. Shame does not consider our gender, ethnicity, relationship status, or socioeconomic standing. No amount of personal success can avoid it. And as Dr. Curt Thompson wrote:

> It doesn't require the breakdown of our mental health to be plagued with it. It only requires that you have a pulse. To be human is to be infected with this phenomenon we call shame.
>
> Shame is something we all experience at some level, more consciously for some than for others. Of course there are the obvious examples that come to mind: times we have felt everything from slight embarrassment to deep humiliation. . . . But many of us carry shame less publicly, often outside the easy view of even some of our closest friends. . . . And our coping strategies have become so automatic that we may be completely unaware of its presence and activity.[1]

For many of us, when shame enters the story, what we tell ourselves is not simply based on our actions (often in the form of "I can't" or "I didn't" statements) but aimed at our inherent value as individuals (for example, "I am" or "I am not" statements). That's because shame infects our beliefs about our identity. In the event of failure or a mistake, shame sinks its teeth deeper than addressing behavior and goes right to attacking identity. Where guilt says, "You made a mistake and need to clean up your mess" (that's obviously healthy!), shame says, "You *are* a mistake."

Shame, you see, is devious. It steers your core beliefs. Perhaps that's why shame wants to hijack the driver's seat of your life and write your story. When shame picks up its pen, the narrative it composes is circular and insidious, like a soul cancer that metastasizes throughout your entire being. It's subtle yet overwhelming, sinister and unrelenting. As Thompson pointed out:

> It is actively, *intentionally,* at work both within and between individuals. Its goal is to disintegrate any and every system it targets, be that one's personal story, a family, marriage, friendship, church, school, community, business or political system. Its power lies in its subtlety and its silence, and it will not be satisfied until all hell breaks loose. Literally.[2]

Therefore, the fight is for the permission to write your story and the battleground is indeed your heart.

In the previous chapter, we talked about the broken spirit and described how shame perpetuates the life of the cycle of pain. In this chapter, then, I want to get under the hood of shame and investigate it afresh. Unquestionably, much has been said about shame in the last several decades, thanks to John Bradshaw's *Healing the Shame That Binds You* from 1988 and the more recent remarkable contributions by the likes of Curt Thompson and Brené Brown.

I'm so thankful for their work. But in the context of this book, where our framework is healing what can never be erased from our lives, I want to explore the angle of shame in relation to our stories: how shame intercepts our roadmaps to wholeness and plots its own roadmap to separateness, isolation, victimhood, and destruction.

And just as we are wired for story, I believe shame thrives in its own story arc, composed of four distinct plot elements: the *moment* of shame (which we will cover in this chapter), followed by the *mode,* the *movement,* and the *maturity* of shame (which we will unpack in chapter 5).

Let's dive in.

THE MOMENT OF SHAME

One working definition of *shame* is the "intensely painful feeling or experience of believing that we are flawed and therefore unworthy of love, belonging, and connection."[3] What was the inciting incident in your life that established this devastating precedent? When did shame first intercept the narrative and attempt to steer you away from connection and wholeness toward independence and isolation? Interestingly, while we encounter shame throughout the course of our lives, my own life experiences motivate me to believe that the inciting incident, the *first* moment of shame that often occurs in our early years, has a profound impact on how we negotiate with life going forward. That was the case for me.

Shame was the embarrassment of staining my new shorts as a little boy. Shame was a sidekick to my inability to fit in among my tall, athletic, gregarious peers in high school. Shame was sinking into the restaurant booth after enduring an onslaught of unsubstantiated accusation from someone I loved and respected. And shame was my mom dying of cancer after I subconsciously and erroneously determined that it was my job to make sure she got healed. Today, as a pastor and coach, I regularly meet with people whose stories of shame play out uniquely but all lead down the same path toward disconnection and isolation. Many of their experiences span their early years to the present day.

How many of the following examples resonate with you?[4]

- Shame showed up in grade school when your parents couldn't afford to give you money for the pizza lunch and you had to bring cold homemade pizza in a brown paper bag instead.

- Shame arrived when your dad was buzzed at your Little League game for the third time that season.
- Shame entered your heart when you overheard your mom tell her friend that she wanted to divorce your dad.
- Shame is sexual addiction, especially when you have a great marriage.
- Shame is being overlooked for the promotion at work for the third time.
- Shame is an autoimmune disease diagnosis.
- Shame is losing your job and having to move in with your parents at age forty.
- Shame is having to shop at the secondhand store for your kids' clothing when you were once the person who regularly donated to that same store.
- Shame is going to the second baby shower this month after having been told you'll never be able to conceive naturally.
- Shame is sexual dysfunction as a young, newly married person.
- Shame is being a size 14 when all your friends are a size 4.
- Shame is rejection in another relationship, not because of a character flaw but seemingly because of a physical characteristic you cannot change.

And as a result of shame, most people hide and disconnect from others, including their most trusted relationships. Why? Because they believe they are uniquely and fatally flawed—not because of what they have or haven't done but simply because of *who they are.*[5]

But this expression of shame is not new to humanity by any means. It's why I want to explore the first of shame's four plot elements (the moment of shame) through an anthropological lens. For the sake of our application, doing so will involve talking less about what shame *is* than about what shame *does to us* and how it attempts to hijack and rewrite our stories. I believe this approach will not only validate the insidious nature of shame but also prove that its lethal potential is equal to its primitive history in the human race. Because shame is as old as we are, let's explore its roots through the early account of humanity in the book of Genesis.

The Anthropology of Shame

In the beginning, there was no shame, for sin and its consequences had not yet entered the world. In fact, soon after Eve was created out of Adam's rib, the Bible records, "The man and his wife were both naked and were not ashamed."[6] I'm curious why Scripture describes them in these terms. Why not characterize them as being naked and carefree? Or unafraid? Why were they specifically described as being *unashamed*? This begs the question, "What about shame is so primitive to the human experience?"

To explore this issue, I sought the counsel of Dr. Curt Thompson in late 2020 when I first hosted him on my podcast. In our interview, Curt told me that while we don't completely know *why* or *how*, we do know *that* shame is primal. And, he said, we see that shame was already working its way into the story through the conversation between the serpent and Eve, which transpired before any fruit was eaten, because "if it wasn't, the woman would have no reason to be eating fruit in the first place."[7]

As such, early in the narrative of Scripture, I believe we're given a clue that two avenues by which shame establishes a footing in our lives are isolation (separateness) and deception. It was true in the garden[8] and it's true for us today. When we separate ourselves from regular communion with the Lord, the Scriptures, and the safety of wise counsel, we will inevitably lack the discernment to detect a lie at its inception because we haven't maintained a standard of truth by which all arguments, theories, and reasonings are examined.[9] And sadly, when we don't quickly assess and arrest a lie for what it is, we're trapped by it. This was the case for Eve. Here's Genesis 3:1–7:

> The serpent was more crafty than any other beast of the field that the LORD God had made.

He said to the woman, "Did God actually say, 'You shall not eat of any tree in the garden'?" And the woman said to the serpent, "We may eat of the fruit of the trees in the garden, but God said, 'You shall not eat of the fruit of the tree that is in the midst of the garden, neither shall you touch it, lest you die.'" But the serpent said to the woman, "You will not surely die. For God knows that when you eat of it your eyes will be opened, and you will be like God, knowing good and evil." So when the woman *saw* that the tree was good for food, and that it was a *delight* to the eyes, and that the tree was to be desired to make one wise, she took of its fruit and ate, and she also gave some to her husband who was with her, and he ate. Then the *eyes of both were opened,* and *they knew that they were naked.* And they sewed fig leaves together and made themselves loincloths.

Let's unpack this trajectory of events that led to sin, which birthed shame into the human experience:

1. **The Temptation:** The serpent probed Eve, "Did God *actually* say . . . ?" Though Eve was sinless at the time, she was seducible and susceptible to temptation because a human being with free will and a soul has desire. The serpent's inquiry was an attempt to cause Eve to question the Lord's nature. It wasn't about checking the facts. It was about sowing a seed of doubt. The serpent's insinuation was clear: If God was good and kind, why would He restrict her from enjoying the fullness of delight in the garden? Thus, if the serpent could motivate Eve to question the *nature* of the Lord, he would likely succeed in causing her to question the *ways* of the Lord (His direction, commands, and actions). And once she questioned the nature and the ways of the Lord, her heart would be vulnerable to distrust, where she would presumably act in independence and disobey His commands.

Though temptation in and of itself is not sin, it breaks open the door to deception, where we are baited to believe and act on a lie. And when we believe a lie, we empower it to thrive *as if it were truth* in our lives, which results in death. The apostle James reinforced this principle when he said, "Let no one say when he is tempted, 'I am being tempted by God,' for God cannot be tempted with evil, and he himself tempts no one. But each person is tempted when he is *lured and enticed by his own desire.* Then desire when it has conceived gives birth to sin, and sin when it is fully grown brings forth death."[10]

2. **The Consideration:** Temptation doesn't automatically lead to sin and death, except when we believe the inbuilt lie and act on it. But before we believe a lie, we weigh it against what we currently believe to be true. Eve's reply to the serpent's temptation was exactly in this stride; she presented the facts as she had been told: "We may eat of the fruit of the trees in the garden, but God said, 'You shall not eat of the fruit of the tree that is in the midst of the garden, neither shall you touch it, lest you die.' "[11]

3. **The Lie:** The serpent immediately capitalized on the moment and planted the lie. It's important to understand that the strength of any good lie relies on a measure of truth. Cunningly, the serpent replied, "You will not surely die. For God knows that when you eat of it your eyes will be opened, and you will be like God, knowing good and evil."[12] In other words, *Eve, you must have misunderstood God. If He loves you, why would He withhold anything good from you?* The serpent's devious rationale resonated with Eve in such a way that she believed and acted on the lie.

4. **The Moment of Shame:** As a result of their sin, Adam's and Eve's eyes were opened, and they knew they were na-

ked. Their innocence before the Lord and before each other was replaced by guilt and shame. Sin opened the door for shame to manifest itself in all of humanity.

5. **The Cover-up:** In response to their guilt and shame and the awareness of their nakedness, "they sewed fig leaves together and made themselves loincloths."[13] And having covered themselves through their own effort toward self-protection, they hid.

Quite obviously, shame is one of the most primitive emotions known to the human race, and we all experience it today. But shame's potency is more insidious than what we might typically ascribe to an emotion. Thompson said, "This phenomenon is the *primary tool that evil leverages,* out of which emerges everything that we would call sin."[14] Simply stated, because of sin, shame exists and has the potential to make us cynical and bitter. It has the capacity to cripple our potential. And left alone, it will make us sick.

Therefore, I wholeheartedly believe that because shame is a dominant driver in keeping us stuck in the cycle of pain, we need to expose and eradicate shame at the root level—the inciting moment when the seed is planted. As we learned in the last chapter, a person whose spirit is broken will view life's adversity through a lens of defeat and despair, seeing their mistakes and missed opportunities as an indictment on their identity. To bring application to this theory, let's revisit one of my earliest experiences with shame and explore how a planted seed had the potential to grow and affect my life going forward.

ANALYZING THE SHORTS INCIDENT

In an effort to clearly identify the development and influence shame had on my life, take a look at how my early-in-life moment of shame metastasized and thus dominated my soul into young adulthood:

1. **The Inciting Incident:** As I mentioned, when I was a young boy, I accidentally stepped on a piece of fruit while walking down a sidewalk with a trusted adult, and the juice from the fruit squirted onto my clean shorts. Though it wasn't a big deal in the grand scheme of things, my immediate response was embarrassment, which disarmed me and made me vulnerable to what came next: the seed of shame.

2. **The Seed of Shame:** The person's response not only validated my embarrassment but also provoked a faulty belief statement about my identity. She shouted, "How could you be so blind? You have nothing else to wear! *You're useless!* As smart as you are, why are you *so stupid* sometimes? This is your fault and you're going to have to *fix this yourself*!" Though stepping on the fruit was a simple accident, my young, impressionable heart received the words from someone I trusted and believed as an indictment of my inherent value. I hadn't yet developed the emotional maturity to understand her callous words as an inappropriate overextension of frustration and anger about an accident and separate them from the truth about my safety and belonging as a child. And sadly, because I hid from the embarrassment and shame of that situation and didn't bring it to my parents until much later, the seed of shame was planted, and it seized the opportunity to drive my subconscious narrative through my formative years. This is essentially a case study on the power of a believed lie to steer our lives. Had a minor, fixable accident occurred? Yes. Was I useless and stupid? No. But because I *believed* those caustic words, "I am useless and stupid" became a subconscious narrative (false identity) from which I lived as if it were really true.

3. **The Outgrowth of Shame:** As simple as that example may seem, the compounded adverse circumstances in my life

validated the twisted shame narrative I was believing. Fundamentally, no matter what people told me, the life I saw plainly with my eyes and experienced each day seemed to prove that I would never be safe unless I made my life small and insular. As I already shared, my life throughout my teenage and young adult years then became motivated by perfectionism, self-protection, and insecurity just to stay afloat and to cope with the false identity of "I am useless and stupid." Though the cycle was devastating and utterly dysfunctional, I didn't know anything different. Worst of all, this performance-driven shame narrative convinced me that it was my job to make sure my mom didn't die.

4. **The Soul Ruled by Shame:** Thus, the dominant driver in my life was the identity of an orphan—substantiated by the subconscious belief that I was useless and stupid. It drove me into a continual uphill climb where I worked (and worked) and strived (and strived) for worth, connection, and belonging.

And it all began with a tiny seed of a lie that was left to settle and germinate in my soul until it matured into something I called "true," even though my *true* was far from *the truth*. While my shorts incident was really nothing to lose sleep over (because the shorts were either washed or replaced), it was the Trojan horse by which a shame-invoking incident implanted a lie, which then birthed a false identity and steered my life. Think of nearly any circumstance from your own life that evoked a similar response. The circumstance might be difficult or even devastating. But below the surface, the Enemy has used it as a container for shame to deliver faulty information about who you are and whose you are.

Earlier in the chapter, I posed the question "What about shame is so primitive to the human experience?" Why is shame so insidious and effective? Well, having spent some time on the subject with you thus far, I want to share this working theory: *The strength of shame is that it hooks itself to our identity.* And whatever has our identity has our beliefs. Whatever has our beliefs has our thoughts. Whatever has our thoughts has the affections of our hearts. And whatever has our affections has our focus and thus the motivation and direction for our lives, because whatever has the most influence over us *has us.* This is why psychological, subjective, toxic shame must be called out for what it is: a thief and a killer. If the Enemy of our souls can use shame to inform our identities, we will live as orphans who are motivated to self-protect and self-promote, not as adopted children of a King who are called "more than conquerors"[15] and whose mandate is to be fruitful, co-create, and extend the kingdom of God here on the earth.

> The strength of shame is that it hooks itself to our identity.

Under shame's influence, instead of pursuing truth and freedom through intimacy with the Lord, where we willingly pray, "Search me, O God, and know my heart! Try me and know my thoughts,"[16] we will stand at a distance even from the One who knit us together in our mother's womb.[17] We will put on a front, because coming to Him in our shame is too great a risk of additional humiliation. And when He says, "Come to Me, all you who labor and are heavy-laden and overburdened,"[18] we will run away. It is this very shame that gives life to our broken spirits and keeps us stuck in a perpetual state of defeat and despair.

For more than thirty years, researchers, psychologists, and medical professionals more qualified than I to speak on this subject have contributed remarkable wisdom to our understanding of shame and our ability to develop resilience against it. Yet our persistent communal struggle with shame appears to demonstrate why secular humanism and self-help strategies at their best—as helpful as they are to provide strategies to change our *behavior*—can never transform our *hearts* and thus change our lives.

PERSONALIZE IT

THE POINT

When shame enters our stories, what we tell ourselves is based not simply on our actions but rather on our inherent individual value. That's because shame infects our beliefs about our identity.

THE PROMPT

When did shame first intercept your life and attempt to steer you away from connection and wholeness and instead toward independence and isolation? Can you describe the event or experience? What happened?

THE POSTURE

Frame one of your pivotal experiences with shame (your moment of shame) against my personal analysis of the shorts incident. Walk your experience through the four stages I described. Oftentimes, when we see issues and patterns of dysfunction clearly, we can deal with them most effectively.

THE PRAYER

Lord, I know that shame gains access to my heart through isolation and deception. What lies have I believed and thus empowered to dominate my life? I want to deal with them now in truth. Also, Father, please heal my tentativeness toward You. Shame causes me to hide, and I don't want to hide any longer. I reject superficiality in Jesus's name. I want to live in the light and life of Your presence. Amen.

FIVE

HOW SHAME THRIVES

Everything within me wants to show my best
"pretend self" to both other people and God.
This is my false self—the self of my own making.
This self can never be transformed, because it is
never willing to receive love in vulnerability.

—DAVID G. BENNER, *Surrender to Love*

Having established a foundation for the inciting moments of
shame and an understanding about why unmitigated early experiences
of shame can metastasize throughout the narratives of our
existence, let's dive even deeper and look at the second major plot
element in this story: the *mode* of shame. While shame is complex
in its reach, I believe it is helpful to describe the mode (or method)
of shame as an expression of either self-protection or self-promotion.[1]
In other words, shame causes us to either become
reclusive and hide or assert ourselves in an overt, prideful, and
often insecure manner to gain ground and mark our territory. In
both cases, we are motivated by a false identity kept alive by a root
of fear (the absence of perfect love), which informs a lack of trust
and thus refuses obedience to the ways of the Lord.

In the creation story, sin led to shame, which motivated Adam
and Eve to hide. Genesis 3:8–11 describes the scene:

They heard the sound of the LORD God walking in the garden
in the cool of the day, and the man and his wife *hid*

themselves from the presence of the LORD God among the trees of the garden. But the LORD God called to the man and said to him, "*Where are you?*" And he said, "I heard the sound of you in the garden, and *I was afraid,* because I was naked, and I hid myself." He said, "Who told you that you were naked? Have you eaten of the tree of which I commanded you not to eat?"

Take a closer look at the interaction. Do you think the Lord was asking Adam where he was because He didn't know his location? Certainly not. God is omniscient and omnipresent. Instead, He was asking Adam to tell the truth about the location of his soul, which was now set in fear and shame. Adam's response confirms this: "I was afraid, because I was naked, and I hid myself." And like Adam, many of us hide in our shame where, instead of connection and belonging, even our most trusted relationships are defined by disconnection and a lack of intimacy.

Undeniably, shame thrives in secrecy.[2] When we are under shame's influence, superficial is safe. We hold people at a proverbial arm's length from our hearts because we fear two things: rejection and repeated pain. Because intimacy gives another person access to see the reality of who we are, we fear that if they deem us "too much" or "too broken," they will walk away just like others have in the past. Or we fear that more pain will be inflicted because a person's level of access to our heart is the level by which they can hurt us. Is this fear motivation understandable? Sure. But is it healthy? No.

The fingerprints of the Enemy are categorically *secrecy* and *shame,*[3] and when we are influenced by either (or both), we will remain stuck in the cycle of pain and, worse, feed our broken spirits, giving way to lives characterized by defeat. Moreover, the soul imbued with shame feasts on blame as a countertactic for the crisis unfolding within, and it shuns the need for personal responsibility. Remember Adam's response to the Lord's inquiry? He said, "The woman whom you gave to be with me, she gave me fruit of the tree, and I ate."[4] Eve's response was no different, shifting the blame away from herself: "The serpent deceived me, and I ate."[5]

Now, the reflexive drive to hide ourselves after experiencing shame also involves concealing our vulnerability, shame, and sense of disgrace. We often do so by cloaking our souls with good performance and the approval of others—masking our insecurity with charisma, perfectionism, false humility, and even victimhood. That was my experience. But this self-protective response to shame is nothing new in our anthropology. Let's go back to the garden, right after Adam and Eve ate of the forbidden fruit and just before they hid from the Lord. Genesis 3:7 says, "The eyes of both were opened, and they knew that they were naked. And they *sewed fig leaves together* and *made themselves loincloths.*" Adam and Eve were created in the image and likeness of God, and His likeness is covered with light as a garment.[6] So were they until the onset of sin, which was the exact moment when they noticed their nakedness.[7] Thus, their loincloths were made from their own effort.

And like our predecessors, our best efforts to clothe, protect, and hide ourselves will never remedy the crisis of shame within. It is in this insular posture of self-consciousness that we are vulnerable to deception. If the already-defeated Enemy of our souls can distract, discourage, and deceive us by leveraging shame to rewrite our stories, we will inevitably isolate ourselves from the Vine, telling ourselves, *If He loved me, this situation wouldn't have happened.* And then, just like Adam and Eve became sidetracked from God's command to "be fruitful and multiply and fill the earth and subdue it,"[8] instead of stewarding our kingdom purpose, we will spend our days self-focused and living a false identity to compensate for the lack of purpose, protection, and power that obeying the Lord's commands and staying connected to His presence would have provided. Staying tethered to truth through humility before the Lord is a key difference between the transformation He performs *with our willing partnership* and the self-healing narrative so popular in our humanistic culture.

As I've already stated, whatever adversity or loss you face, the underlying fight is for the right to craft your story either as more than a conqueror[9] or as a victim. The choice is yours. Will you partner with the Holy Spirit for transformation that lifts you out of the ashes of your circumstances and beyond the limitations of your human condition? Or will you choose defeat and victimhood?

I don't intend to be harsh, but I do intend to be clear. Though this is challenging, it is not complicated. In view of eternity, this life is short, and we are stewards of it. And someday, we will give an account of our stewardship to the Lord.[10] Likewise, because the Enemy knows we have a choice in the matter, his method of attack is both crafty and calculated.[11] As he subtly leverages our emotions and thoughts, shame has an open door to dominate our neurophysiology. Through our destructive rumination, neuroplasticity will work in an unproductive, toxic manner, creating hardwired neural pathways that lead to harmful behaviors and unfavorable outcomes that render us stuck as victims of life.

> Through our destructive rumination, neuroplasticity will work in an unproductive, toxic manner, creating hardwired neural pathways that lead to harmful behaviors and unfavorable outcomes that render us stuck as victims of life.

This is the basis for Hebb's axiom (named for neuropsychologist Donald Hebb), which says that "neurons that fire together wire together." Commenting on this theory, Dr. Curt Thompson explained, "In essence, the more we practice activating particular neural networks, the [easier] they are to activate, and the more permanent they become in the brain."[12]

As we will discuss later in the book, this is why renewing our minds (auditing our thoughts) according to the truth of God's Word on a regular basis is an absolutely critical practice. You see, where there is shame, there is an underlying root of fear. And where there is a root of fear, perfect love has not matured in our lives.[13] That's why we easily move toward independence and self-creation, toward self-consciousness and disconnection. Everything in life comes from a motivation of either fear or love. *That's it.* So, where there is perfect love, there is trust. And where trust is found, the fruit of transformation, quick obedience, and intimacy abounds in our lives.

> Everything in life comes from a motivation of either fear or love. *That's it.*

Sadly, however, self-protection and self-promotion have become as familiar to many of us as our favorite sweatshirts. And when they become our default responses to life, the third plot element, the *movement* of shame, enters the picture.

THE MOVEMENT OF SHAME

As shame metastasizes, it affects our spirits, souls, and bodies. In other words, not only does shame cause us to think in a certain way, but the emotion involved also touches our physiology and incites powerful physical sensations in our bodies. To illustrate this point, I'll share the results of a case study I conducted. Recently, I surveyed a few hundred people and asked a simple question: "When you experience shame, what does it feel like in your body?" The responses were consistent and profound:

"Tightening in my chest, making it hard to breathe"
"Heart racing, head spinning"
"Literal pain in my heart"
"A pit in my stomach"
"Heaviness (or weight) on my chest"
"Pressure all around my neck and chest"
"Brain feels offline"
"Numbness in heart and chest, nauseous"
"Heavy, like I want to crawl out of my skin"
"Anxiety in my chest"

Confirming the responses I compiled above, a study conducted by Finnish researchers found that emotions do affect our bodies in consistent patterns. Across five experiments, a group of 701 participants "were shown two silhouettes of bodies alongside emotional words, stories, movies, or facial expressions. They were asked to color the bodily regions whose activity they felt increasing or decreasing while viewing each stimulus. Different emotions were *consistently associated* with statistically separable bodily sensation maps across experiments."[14]

Where did shame show up on the topographical tool? Precisely where my respondents indicated: the head, neck, chest, and stomach. Interestingly, a journalist from *The Atlantic* pointed out that "the correlations between the subjects' different body maps were strong—above .71 for each of the different stimuli (words, stories, and movies). Speakers of Taiwanese, Finnish, and Swedish drew similar body maps, suggesting that the sensations are not limited to a given language."[15] So what does that mean? The researchers concluded that the subjective results were quite similar across many demographics: "Emotional feelings are associated with discrete, yet partially overlapping maps of bodily sensations, which could be at the core of the emotional experience."[16]

In other words, our emotions influence our bodies so much that, as one of my respondents indicated, the presence of shame can make many of us feel like our brains are "offline." And it is this subjective description that intrigues me to further explore possible inferences. Earlier, we considered the mode of shame manifesting as self-protection or self-promotion, both of which are emotionally driven reactions. Whereas the emotion of guilt is most often associated with an action, behavior, or thing outside oneself, the emotion of shame is directly related to one's identity.[17]

I want to make sure you understand the influence of shame on our spirits, souls, and bodies, so allow me to run a thread through the logic we're constructing. Shame is connected to the limbic system in the brain (otherwise known as "the survival brain"), which steers the autonomic nervous system's fight-or-flight responses[18] to stressful situations and is the seat of our emotions and subconscious narratives. So, when shame begins to spiral or attack, higher-level brain activity in the prefrontal cortex (the brain structure that performs executive functions; that is, where we make decisions, reason, and rationalize logically) is less active and gives way to one conquest: survival.[19] And that's exactly why shame causes us to hide.

Validating this idea, Heidi L. Dempsey, a psychology professor at Jackson State University, wrote that shame is "associated with avoidance behaviors such as hiding one's face, collapsing of the body, slumping, or gaze aversion. Shame action tendencies also revolve around expressions of *inadequacy, defectiveness,* wishing to hide or escape, wanting to save face, and wanting to know that the other person does not view him/her as a lesser person."[20]

Consider again the severity of shame based on this statement. Essentially, the inadequacy and defectiveness associated with shame points not to behavior but to identity. And when the false identity of "inadequate and defective"—or in my case "useless and stupid"—drives our subconscious narratives, we outwork life from an insecure disposition where our efforts are an uphill climb just to fit in with others and to compensate for our perceived lack and incompetence.

That's why we costume our souls with perfectionism and victimhood. *That's* why we camouflage our personalities instead of offering the world the uniqueness of our design. *That's* why we self-promote in an overt and insecure manner. And instead of pursuing belonging and connection with safe people, *that's* why we hide, disconnect, and isolate.

Can you see it now? Do you see why shame, unlike guilt, is so lethal? Do you recognize it as the lifeblood of the broken spirit that crashes our potential and renders us defeated in life? Do you see how the Enemy would leverage a tool like shame to distract us from stewarding our kingdom purposes and from living in wholeness? Granted, the Enemy cannot thwart or defeat the eternal purposes of the Lord, for God's kingdom is unstoppable. But the Enemy *can* influence us to the extent that when we are baited by temptation and believe a lie, we're more easily inclined to allow destructive mindsets to be established and to make choices that lead us down paths of defeat. As a result, we turn from our kingdom purposes and live self-conscious and reactionary lives as victims confined to the human condition, instead of walking uprightly in purity and power as the Father's sons and daughters here on earth.

This is why I cannot discuss shame from the perspective of self-help alone. The implications are far too great. In our pursuit of healing from the life experiences we cannot erase, we must maintain an eternal perspective in light of our adoption to sonship.[21] Otherwise, we put religious dressings on humanistic self-help strategies, rise no higher than behavior modification, and totally miss out on the transformation of our spirits, souls, and bodies, not through our own efforts, but by the Holy Spirit's power at work in our willing hearts.

> In our pursuit of healing from the life experiences we cannot erase, we must maintain an eternal perspective in light of our adoption to sonship. Otherwise, we put religious dressings on humanistic self-help strategies, rise no higher than behavior modification, and totally miss out on the transformation of our spirits, souls, and bodies, not through our own efforts, but by the Holy Spirit's power at work in our willing hearts.

Most notably, the absence of transformation is what lays the welcome mat for the fourth plot element: the *maturity* of shame.

THE MATURITY OF SHAME

All of us will experience moments of shame throughout the course of life. For the most part, we move through them largely unscathed. But if shame settles and matures into our identities by winning the fight to write our stories, who do we *become*? What is the subconscious "I am" false determination we receive and then live from? "I am a mistake"? "I am broken and unlovable"? "I'm not worthy of interpersonal connection and belonging"?[22] As you well know, mine was "I am useless and stupid."

And after shame influences our identities, what becomes of our personalities and temperaments? Do we become cynical? Bitter? Perhaps indignant, isolated, and insignificant? Intolerant and insecure? I believe all these descriptors are probable outcomes if early, unhealed experiences of shame plant their roots deeply into our hearts, fortify our broken spirits, and compromise our relationships, health, and life potential. Simply stated, therefore, if transformation is for the integration of our spirits, souls, and bodies, shame is for their disintegration and fragmentation.

> If transformation is for the integration of our spirits, souls, and bodies, shame is for their disintegration and fragmentation.

Consequently, in light of the relation between shame's activity in sustaining a broken spirit and the broader perspective I've shared about our eternal purposes and callings from the Lord (which shame seeks to hijack), we must consider yet another aspect of shame. I believe one of the greatest threats that mature, well-formed shame poses is not that we will someday blow up our lives through reckless living; it is that we will live idly and do *nothing* with our lives, that we will bury our talents and abdicate our stewardship to multiply what the Lord has given us to manage.

Understand that when shame has signed, sealed, and delivered the identity "You are useless and stupid," and we believe and receive it as truth even though it is a blatant lie, our creativity and drive to add value to the world are stunted. Why? Because a person who believes they are useless and stupid *at their core* not only feels that they have nothing to contribute, but they also react by living in isolation—away from the community of believers where the light of truth can destroy lies through the power of vulnerability, belonging, and the presence of the Holy Spirit.

MOVING FORWARD THROUGH SHAME TO TRANSFORMATION

Moving forward through shame to transformation will not happen by chance. As I stated in chapter 2, good information alone won't change our lives. Thus, moving beyond shame requires a teachable spirit and a willingness to confront one's own dysfunction. It necessitates a regular commitment to wrestle with issues of the heart through vulnerability before the Lord and one's trusted community, as well as the development (and regular practice) of skills like shame resilience.

Brené Brown's extensive research through the University of Houston led to four key components of developing shame resilience:

"Recognizing shame and understanding its triggers." The question to begin the process is, "Can you physically recognize when you're in the grip of shame, name it, feel your way through it, and figure out what messages and expectations triggered it?"

"Practicing critical awareness." Regarding this step, Brown inquires, "Can you reality-check the messages and expectations that are driving your shame? Are they realistic? Attainable? Are they what you want to be or what you think others need or want from you?"

"Reaching out." If shame causes us to hide and isolate, vulnerability in community promotes healing. This is why Brown probes, "Are you owning and sharing your story?"

"Speaking shame." Can we speak freely about our experiences with shame among a community of safe people? Shame thrives where isolation abounds, for "silence, secrecy, and judgment fuel shame."[23]

Brown says these four steps "rarely happen in this order—they just all need to happen for us to develop resilience to shame."[24]

But as helpful as these steps are, as disciples of Jesus whose hearts are to be directed toward the priorities and values of God's kingdom, we must not stop our pursuit of healing at the limits of our minds and behavior. Nor should we even engage with a practice that "from the standpoint of naturalistic evolution . . . merely functions as a moderator of human interactions."[25] To do so would grossly overlook a critical understanding about the greater narrative of humanity and our individual purposes in God's eternal plan, let alone insinuate that secular humanism and the wisdom of this age hold *any* meaningful stake in our healing journeys. Instead, through the Scriptures, by the power of the Holy Spirit, and in a safe and trusted community of other believers, we are invited into a process of *transformation* in the deepest parts of our beings: the human spirit. And transformation requires vulnerability.

The Invitation to Vulnerability

Perhaps when we hear the word *vulnerability* (or *vulnerable*), we associate it with life experiences such as being accused of wrongdoing, engaging in difficult conversations, or making mistakes in front of others and subsequently feeling embarrassed. "This," as Thompson pointed out, "is not an inaccurate description of what it means to feel vulnerable, but it is not complete. In reality, vulnerability is not something we choose or that is true in a given moment, while the rest of the time it is not. Rather, it is something we *are*. . . . To be human *is* to be vulnerable."[26]

Therefore, a clear picture of vulnerability is embodied in the Genesis account of creation where Adam and Eve "were both naked and were not ashamed."[27] And what a picture that is to us—or rather an invitation. Our humble vulnerability before the Lord and before our community, which extricates the root of shame from our souls, requires nakedness. It requires a decided unwillingness to clothe ourselves in a false identity of pretense, pride, self-protection, insecurity, perfectionism, performance, or anything that would inhibit a full view of who we really are, brokenness and all.

Certainly, this level of vulnerability is not easy. Psychologist and author David Benner explained why vulnerability is such a challenge:

> Everything within me wants to show my best "pretend self" to both other people and God. This is my false self—the self of my own making. This self can never be transformed, because it is never willing to receive love in vulnerability. When this pretend self receives love, it simply becomes stronger and I am even more deeply in bondage to my false ways of living.
>
> Both popular psychology and spirituality—even popular Christian spirituality—tend to reinforce this false self by playing to our deep-seated belief in self-improvement.[28]

This is precisely why the deeper work of healing the broken, unredeemed narratives about our painful life experiences requires transformation, not self-help or self-healing, and why forging a roadmap to wholeness requires us to forsake the false. Remember David's words from Psalm 24? He wrote,

> Who shall ascend the hill of the LORD?
>   And who shall stand in his holy place?
> He who has clean hands and a pure heart,
>   who does not lift up his soul to what is false
>   and does not swear deceitfully.[29]

You see, this idea of designing our roadmaps to wholeness isn't about self-satisfaction or comfort, even though when we walk in the ways of the Lord, we are positioned for blessing. And healing what we can't erase isn't about achieving a state of utopia. That's self-help and secular humanism with a Christian veneer.

On the contrary, charting our course to wholeness is about the transformation of our spirits, souls, and bodies so that we may ascend the mountain of the Lord with clean hands and pure hearts. Moreover, it's so that we may steward the lives we have been given with excellence and authority for the glory of the Lord and the expansion of His kingdom.

Benner validated this notion when he wrote,

> The life and message of Jesus stand diametrically opposed to such efforts at self-improvement. Jesus did not come to encourage our self-transformation schemes. He understood that rather than longing to receive his love in an undefended state, what we really want is to manipulate God to accept us in our false and defended ways of being. If only he would do this, we could remain unaware of just how desperately we need real love.[30]

When we learn how to abide in God's perfect love that drives out every trace of fear (a refuge of His presence where trust and obedience remain), the root of shame—that compulsive drive to hide in self-protection and assert ourselves in pride and insecurity—will be broken.

Shame's lethal and destructive nature once caused us to be motivated by self-preservation and isolation. But now the Author and Finisher of our faith calls us to Himself, where everything once unexposed must come into the light of His presence, to receive healing. He is the One who brings complete meaning to the fragmentation of our experiences.

And it gets better. Not only does the Lord redeem our past, but He also restores and rebuilds what was lost. Having been bound up and restored, we are called "oaks of righteousness" in our generation,[31] those whom He uses to bring healing and restoration to others. "Instead of your shame," Isaiah prophesied, "there shall be a double portion; instead of dishonor they shall rejoice in their lot; therefore in their land they shall possess a double portion; they shall have everlasting joy."[32]

So, lift up the eyes of your heart today. Your salvation comes not from within but from above. He has called you by name and has lifted you up out of the ashes. Now, will you stand up and walk with Him? Will you follow Him on this spiritual journey toward transformation?

My prayer is that you will vehemently deny shame (or any self-preserving, fear-formed obstacle) the privilege of directing your life another day. And you'll do this not by striving but by surrender.

PERSONALIZE IT

THE POINT

Shame thrives in secrecy and often manifests in self-protection or self-promotion. It affects us in spirit, soul, and body. And left unchecked, shame settles and matures into our identities by winning the fight to write our stories.

THE PROMPT

When you experience shame, what does it feel like in your body? Also, because shame thrives in secrecy, what long-hidden secrets do you need to bring into the light of God's presence and within a community of safe people? Lastly, because of shame's influence in your life, what is the subconscious "I am" false determination you received and have lived from?

THE POSTURE

How will you position yourself this week to begin to move forward through shame toward transformation? To learn and apply the skills of shame resilience in your life? This will require priority in your calendar, and it will not be a onetime event. Please schedule time with a counselor; your pastor; or another trusted, spiritually mature, emotionally intelligent mentor. Discuss with them your answers regarding your moment, mode, movement, and maturity of shame. Remember that transformation does not happen in a day. It happens *daily.*

THE PRAYER

Lord, I now understand that moving forward through shame requires a teachable spirit and a willingness to confront my own dysfunction. Give me the grace to do just that each and every day. I also ask that You help me discern the safe, mature people to whom I can be vulnerable. I'm done hiding. I'm done pretending. And I'm done wearing the mask of self-protection and self-promotion. You can have my heart—all of it. In Jesus's mighty name I pray. Amen.

SIX

THE ART OF SURRENDER

The greatness of a man's power is the measure
of his surrender.

—J. WILBUR CHAPMAN

Most Wednesday nights for the past several years, I've met with an incredible man named Dave. Our meeting is one of those immovable commitments—unless something unexpected or urgent arises, nothing interferes with our time together. It's part mentoring and part fellowship, though most of our time is spent studying and talking about the Word of God.

I've given him (and his co-counselor wife, Connie) access to speak into every area of my life, and they do. But as life-giving and vital as their relationship is to me today, it began on the heels of my internal crisis. Our first session together came at the behest of mutual friends who recommended I meet with Dave and Connie for counseling.

Desperate as I was for help but lacking the awareness of exactly *what* I needed, I thought anything was worth a shot. Stuck in the exact cycle of pain we discussed in chapter 3, my broken spirit, aching for resuscitation, was met with stability, wisdom, and great compassion in their presence. For the first time in over a decade, I felt safe enough to drop my self-protective armor. I was exhausted and knew I couldn't carry the weight anymore. And as I let my guard down in that first meeting, I fell apart.

With careful attention, they didn't respond with many words, because words weren't needed. Instead, I just needed presence, and presence is what I received. Everyone needs a Dave and Connie in their lives.

Over the next few months, they led me through a process of both grief counseling and inner healing. It was hard. It was confrontational. But I didn't need sympathy anymore. I needed my life transformed. Thankfully, because I was raised in a stable home by incredible parents, my foundation was solid. But rebuilding and restoring my life after significant traumatic losses would first require deconstructing the walls I had put up over the last several years.

This process reminds me of what Paul wrote in 2 Corinthians 10:3–5: "Though we walk in the flesh, we are not waging war according to the flesh. For the weapons of our warfare are not of the flesh but have divine power to destroy strongholds. We destroy arguments and every lofty opinion raised against the knowledge of God, and take every thought captive to obey Christ." The Amplified Bible Classic Edition translates verse 5 this way: "[Inasmuch as we] refute arguments and theories and reasonings and every proud and lofty thing that sets itself up against the [true] knowledge of God; and we lead every thought and purpose away captive into the obedience of Christ (the Messiah, the Anointed One)." Though I had plenty of seemingly justifiable arguments, theories, and reasons for my state of being, each represented a brick that built the walls of self-protection over my heart. So, if transformation was indeed my aim, surrender was my first necessary initiative.

In my earliest sessions with Dave and Connie, surrender looked like giving up self-preservation and control—loosening my grip on the safe, small life I had compulsively constructed. But over time, surrender took on a new form. Instead of giving *up*, surrender became about giving *in* to a process of confrontation that would lead to transformation of my life from the inside out. And the same will be true for you too. In chapter 3, we learned that the cycle of pain, through isolation, disconnects us from the Vine and builds walls around our hearts. In this chapter, we'll learn that the process of surrender that leads to transformation is about tearing down those hard-hearted walls and reconnecting to the Vine.

As for you, I want you to know with all sincerity that no one who has your best interest at heart (including the Lord) invalidates the pain, loss, abuse, trauma, or disappointment you've experienced. But like me, you must not allow a *season* of life to write the *story* of your life. Fear is designed to make things stop,[1] specifically forward progress in life.

> You must not allow a *season* of life to write the *story* of your life.

So, the question I want you to honestly answer today is this: Do you want to be free? Do you really *want* to deal with what you *need* to in order to live a life characterized by transformation and wholeness? The Holy Spirit lovingly and willingly meets us where we are, right in the middle of our pain and sorrow, and without hesitation in our doubt and despair. But we have to choose to partner with Him in this process of transformation. The question is, Will we? Will *you*? The day you decide that the pain of regret is greater than the pain of change is the day you'll take a first step toward the process of transformation to wholeness.[2] And as a reminder, none of us can change ourselves from the inside out. Only the power of the Holy Spirit working in us can enact systemic change. But we can—and we *must*—position ourselves to receive His dynamic, thorough work of healing by surrendering our self-protection, isolation, shame, blame, and broken spirits to Him.

When those walls around your heart fall and you reattach to the Vine, transformation is inevitable. That was indeed the situation for a blind beggar named Bartimaeus, whose story in Mark 10 serves as a case study about freedom and transformation in the face of a formidable personal challenge.

Bartimaeus sat on the roadside in Jericho each day, cloaked in an outer garment that gave legitimacy to his need and arguably provided him with a measure of physical security. Though there was no denying his condition, he was unwilling to find sufficiency and identity in his deficiency. One day, he heard commotion and sensed that Jesus and His disciples were nearby. Bartimaeus decided not another day would pass without experiencing the healing he knew was his, so he put a desperate demand on the moment for his breakthrough. Mark 10:47 captures his impassioned cry: "Jesus, Son of David, have pity and mercy on me [now]!" (AMPC). Verse 48 continues, "Many severely censured and reproved him, telling him to keep still, but he kept on shouting out all the more, You Son of David, have pity and mercy on me [now]!"

No doubt, Jesus's disciples viewed his pleas as an interruption to the procession, but Bartimaeus pressed on amid the rebukes of the crowd. Verse 49 says, "Jesus stopped and said, Call him. And they called the blind man, telling him, Take courage! Get up! He is calling you." The next moment was pivotal: "Throwing off his outer garment," the gospel writer recorded, "he leaped up and came to Jesus."[3] Jesus then asked him, "What do you want Me to do for you? And the blind man said to Him, Master, let me receive my sight. And Jesus said to him, Go your way; your faith has healed you. And at once he received his sight and accompanied Jesus on the road."[4]

Bartimaeus's unique story of transformation illuminates three shared movements that will establish guidance for our own pursuit of freedom.

SURRENDER REQUIRES TRUTH

Surrendering to a process of transformation first requires truth and transparency on the inside. Freedom and healing come not to the person we're pretending to be but to the person we are today. The hidden, broken places of our hearts must be unearthed and brought into the light of the Holy Spirit's presence if we desire and expect any measure of sustainable healing in life. We must lay every disappointment, every doubt, and every ounce of distrust before His feet in absolute truth. He already knows the truth, for He *is* the truth.

> Freedom and healing come not to the person we're pretending to be but to the person we are today.

Thus, the invitation is offered to you and me: Will we exchange our true experiences, as traumatic as they were, for the Truth that will set us free? This is the power of confession. I'll illustrate my point with a story.

My good friend and mentor Jamie Winship was a police officer in the 1980s. He often explains that when he arrested someone, he would sit them down and ask for a confession. But in doing so, he wasn't seeking an apology; he was asking for an honest acknowledgment of truth, a true statement about what happened.[5] So it is with us. No matter the complexity or duration of the circumstances in which we find ourselves, our transformation will take shape in the same manner—when we come to the Lord in full truth. About this, Jamie wrote, "Confession is telling God the truth about what you really believe about him, yourself, and others. It's the greatest act, a sacrament. God loves honest confession. Confession is the beginning of genuine transformation."[6]

When we think about the word *confession,* we usually attribute to it personal remorse about the way we acted in a particular situation. And while that's valid and appropriate, it's not a complete picture. The Greek word for "confess" is *homologeō,* which means "to say the same thing as." But secondary definitions of the word include "not to deny; to profess; to declare openly, speak out freely."[7] What is that? It's truth telling that leads us to freedom. Truth isn't simply an intellectual ascent whereby we come to a correct logical conclusion about a matter. The point of truth is freedom. Jesus said to His disciples in John 8:31–32, "If you abide in my word, you are truly my disciples, and you will know the truth, and the truth will set you free."

Let's reference the case study I shared earlier for a closer look at how truth catalyzes transformation. Bartimaeus could have hidden within the throng of people surrounding Jesus. But in the face of his blindness, he roused himself from hiddenness and isolation and chose to present his true condition to the One whose invitation to experience truth would set him free. This was expressed in his unabashed cry for help: "Jesus, Son of David, have mercy on me *now*!" Truth, you see, always emanates from the inside. It has to, because Scripture instructs us to guard our hearts, "for everything [we] do flows" from them.[8]

In Psalm 51:6, which David penned after the prophet Nathan confronted him about his adulterous behavior with Bathsheba,[9] he wrote, "Behold, you delight in truth in the inward being, and you teach me wisdom in the secret heart." Again, when our "true" collides with God's truth, the cords of secrecy, sin, and shame that are suffocating our hearts begin to break and the walls of self-protection start to crumble. Over the months that I worked with Dave and Connie, every time I brought to the Lord a transparent, unfiltered account of my heart's condition—from the fear to the feelings of abandonment and the subsequent drive to preserve my own life—a fresh portion of healing returned to my spirit and soul.

Recently, I experienced another level of freedom. After a series of counseling sessions and time with the Lord, I realized that I had been living under the lie that it was my job to make sure my mom didn't die. And because I had "failed" at my job when she passed away, someone had to bear the consequences—and that person was me. My soul was crushed and my spirit broken, and I believe my body unmasked an autoimmune disease as a result. My internal narrative was "You had one job." So, for the last several years, I have been striving to undo failure that wasn't mine to own in the first place.

Now I want to flip this around to you. Think through the various phases of the cycle of pain from chapter 3. When in your life did you first become disappointed and disillusioned? What event or circumstance caused you to rein in your trust of others, including the Lord? Are you currently motivated to isolate yourself inside your own pain? Are you driven to self-promote in an overtly insecure manner because you feel as though loss has hijacked your hope, identity, and self-worth? Tell the Lord specifically that. Hide nothing. He already knows the thoughts and intentions of your heart, and He desires truth in your inner being. Gone is the safety of your mask. It's time to disrobe from the outer garments of pretense and self-preservation.

Are you wounded? Say to Him, "Here I am, Lord."

Are you afraid? "Here I am, Lord."

Are you cynical? "Here I am, Lord."

Are you hiding in sin and shame? He says to you, "Come out of hiding."

The point is that He will not deal with us in the false. We will talk about identity later in the book, but for now, I'll say this: Two of the most important questions we must reconcile in life are whether we believe we are who He says we are *and* whether we believe He is who He says He is.

In Jeremiah 1:5, the Lord came to Jeremiah and said, "Before I formed you in the womb I knew you, and before you were born I consecrated you; I appointed you a prophet to the nations." Therein, the Lord ascribed identity to Jeremiah.

But Jeremiah's response wasn't congruent with the Lord's intentions. He countered the Lord in verse 6: "Ah, Lord GOD! Behold, I do not know how to speak, for I am only a youth." Even though the Lord called him by name, Jeremiah identified himself according to his circumstance, which was his timidity about his ability and credentials due to his age.

The Lord responded, "Do not say, 'I am only a youth'; for to all to whom I send you, you shall go, and whatever I command you, you shall speak. Do not be afraid of them, for I am with you to deliver you, declares the LORD."[10] What was true about this situation? Jeremiah was young, and he was insecure about that fact. But what was the *truth*? The truth was that the Lord had anointed Jeremiah as a prophet to the nations, and his ability to step into that calling, to embrace his true identity, required him to trust and obey the Lord by submitting his "true" to the Lord's truth. Truth not only empowers us but sets us free to be who He has called us to be, not by our own might but by the Holy Spirit's power at work in our hearts.

Perhaps today you doubt that the Lord will come through with provision and protection for your life because of a series of repeated losses. Tell Him humbly and honestly, "I don't trust that You will be my provider. I'm really afraid to trust You, because I'm more afraid of being let down again."

Does that level of honesty unsettle you? Does it crumple the cute religious packaging with which you've adorned your communication with Him for most of your life? *Good.* I hope it does. He is a perfect, holy God, yes. But He is our Father. And while I don't believe it is wise to ever approach His presence with a spirit of accusation or pride, you must approach Him in truth and honesty.

> Truth not only empowers us but sets us free to be who He has called us to be, not by our own might but by the Holy Spirit's power at work in our hearts.

With a spirit of humility, cast your cares on the Lord once and for all. Lay your burdens down before Him, and wait in His presence. He comforts all who mourn, but mourning requires you to unabashedly face the truth. In Psalm 62:8, the psalmist implores us to "pour out your hearts before Him." Why? Because "God is a refuge for us (a fortress and a high tower)" (AMPC). Here's Jamie Winship on the matter:

> Hiding the truth always makes you a slave. If you will not tell the truth, you're in bondage to the lie, the deception, and the rationalization. Don't apologize for your perceived reality; tell the truth about it. That's confession. Remorse is not repentance.
>
> Confession activates repentance. Repentance is changing the way you think, turning and going a new way. God tells you the truth about who he really is, who you really are, and who your neighbor really is. God's truth empowers you to

believe in a new way, which leads to thinking in a new way, which leads to acting in a new way.[11]

This is so much greater than thinking positively. This is transformation of the heart by the entire renewal of the mind.

Another aspect of truth telling provides not only liberation but also *healing:* the power of confession in community. Who are your people? Seek them out. Involve them in your journey out of darkness and into His marvelous light of healing and transformation.

James wrote about the inherent strength found in confession within community:

> Confess your sins to one another and pray for one another, that you may be healed. The prayer of a righteous person has great power as it is working. Elijah was a man with a nature like ours, and he prayed fervently that it might not rain, and for three years and six months it did not rain on the earth. Then he prayed again, and heaven gave rain, and the earth bore its fruit.[12]

SURRENDER REQUIRES A TRANSFER

The second aspect of surrender in our context is that once we come to the Lord in truth, His truth illuminates the proverbial outer garments draped on our souls that we must discard to move forward in life, just like it was for Bartimaeus. Ours, however, were woven together by ungrieved losses, unresolved disappointments, shame, regret, pride, insecurity, fear, anxiety-led depression, hopelessness, and a deep sense of worthlessness. We've worn them for so long, in fact, that our true identities in Christ are indistinguishable from the self-protective coverings we wear over our hearts every day.

Sadly, for many, the outer garments have become rather comfortable. In His careful eternal wisdom, aware of the freedom we truly desire, Jesus asks this brilliant question in our moment of reckoning: "What do you want Me to do for you?" Remember, this was the exact rhetorical question He asked of me in October 2014. Our omniscient Father knows what we need before we even ask. But what He's really asking is whether we will take responsibility to steward the life we have been given and sever our ties with an identity defined by adversity—to partner with Him and lay aside every encumbrance that seeks to distract us from His ways.

The apostle Paul called us "more than conquerors."[13] That presupposes the fact that we will, like blind Bartimaeus, have something to conquer in this life. Therefore, will you approach Him in truth and exchange your tattered outer garment for a garment of praise? Jesus came, as prophesied by Isaiah, "to grant to those who mourn in Zion—to give them a beautiful headdress instead of ashes, the oil of gladness instead of mourning, the garment of praise instead of a faint spirit; that they may be called oaks of righteousness, the planting of the LORD, that he may be glorified."[14]

And remember David, who after sinning against the Lord, declared, "The sacrifices of God are a broken spirit; a broken and contrite heart, O God, you will not despise."[15] *Your* broken spirit, He will not despise. It may have been conceived by the seed of ungrieved losses, unresolved disappointments, and believed lies. It may have even been birthed by sin or moral failure. That's between you, the Lord, and your community of trusted counselors. And perhaps for years now, you have nurtured it through shame, self-pity, entitlement, cynicism, and bitterness. But today, will you offer it to the Lord? Again, He will not reject it.

The broken, fallow ground of your heart, when tenderized by the Lord, becomes the perfect seedbed from which new life can grow. A heart submitted to the Lord allows what was meant for destruction to be turned for your good and for His glory. Out of the crushing, the pressing, the dark night seasons, the hiddenness, and the loneliness, rich oil and new wine will come forth from your life. The stunning greatness of our God is that even in our darkness and isolation, He is there. Where can we go from His Spirit? Where can we run from His presence?[16] Even the darkness hides nothing from Him.[17]

So the Lord says to you today, "Give Me your heart. *Give Me your broken spirit.* Give Me the defeat and despair. Allow Me to reform you from the inside out. Not a single tear is wasted. I store them in My bottle.[18] And I waste nothing. It is time to break up the fallow ground of your heart that I may rain righteousness on you![19] The water of My Word poured on the dust and dry places from the wilderness seasons of your life forms clay by which I, the Potter, will fashion for Myself a vessel fit for the Master's use.[20] So come out of hiding today. In My presence is fullness of joy. At My right hand are pleasures forevermore."[21] So, *will you?*

SURRENDER REQUIRES TETHERING

Once we come to the Lord in truth and surrender to Him our broken spirits and outer garments of self-protection and shame, we must tether ourselves to Him. In other words, as branches, we must be grafted back into the Vine. As Jesus said,

> Abide in me, and I in you. As the branch cannot bear fruit by itself, unless it abides in the vine, neither can you, unless you abide in me. I am the vine; you are the branches. Whoever abides in me and I in him, he it is that bears much fruit, for apart from me you can do nothing. If anyone does not abide in me he is thrown away like a branch and withers; and the branches are gathered, thrown into the fire, and burned. If you abide in me, and my words abide in you, ask whatever you wish, and it will be done for you.[22]

Interestingly, a branch is grafted back into a vine cut to cut, where the vascular tissues of the branch and the vine are placed against one another, allowing the vine's life-giving nutrients to restore the branch through vital union.[23] And in the same manner, when we expose our wounds to the Wounded Healer, His wounds become our healing. By His stripes, we are indeed healed and made whole.[24]

But transformation doesn't happen in a day; it's not an overnight process. Instead, transformation happens daily. And re-exposing your wounds is risky business for sure. Even riskier, however, is living a dormant and stuck life.

After having thrown off his outer garment, Bartimaeus took action and followed Jesus. The finished work of Jesus Christ on the cross and the power of the Holy Spirit at work in our lives are sufficient to restore us in spirit, soul, and body. Yet transformation from the inside out requires our obedient action in response to God's Word.

Remember the wedding at Cana, the site of Jesus's first public miracle? "Jesus said to the servants, 'Fill the jars with water.' And they filled them up to the brim. And he said to them, 'Now draw some out and take it to the master of the feast.' So they took it."[25] The *servants* had to fill the pots with water before He turned the contents into wine. And I think that resembles our lives in many ways. While Jesus can do a miracle independent of us (and we celebrate that!), *transformation* requires our partnership.

So, today, are you tired and weary? Are self-protection and self-preservation exhausting enough for you to do something about them yet? If so, listen to Jesus. He said, "Come to me, all who labor and are heavy laden, and I will give you rest. Take my yoke upon you, and learn from me, for I am gentle and lowly in heart, and you will find rest for your souls. For my yoke is easy, and my burden is light."[26]

THE NEXT STEP

Come to Him in truth. Lay your burdens down. Throw off your outer garment once and for all. That's your part. Take His yoke, which speaks to direction and pace for life. Graft yourself back onto the Vine, open wounds and all. Relearn trust—trust established not in the certainty of an outcome but in the character and nature of the sovereign One who is "the same yesterday and today and forever,"[27] the One who said He would "never leave you nor forsake you,"[28] no matter what you walk through in life. I know it takes time, but anchor every affection of your heart on Jesus, your living hope. The burden you've been carrying is far too heavy; in fact, it's unnecessary. But because you may have been carrying it for so long, it just feels like "Tuesday," doesn't it? And that's no way to live. So, when will enough be . . . *enough*?

You don't have what it takes to fix or heal yourself. None of us do, and I say that from personal experience. Remember my black binder? How'd that work out for me? *Exactly.* Often, the very things we do to protect ourselves and survive are the things that keep us stuck. Surrender requires truth. Surrender requires a transfer. And surrender requires us to tether ourselves afresh to the Vine.

As Paul prayed for the church in Thessalonica, so I pray for you today these words: "May the God of peace himself sanctify you completely, and may your whole spirit and soul and body be kept blameless at the coming of our Lord Jesus Christ. He who calls you is faithful; he will surely do it."[29] Take courage and get up. He's calling you. He's faithful. And He will surely do it.

Having explored the art of surrender before the Lord, the next inescapable experience through which we must traverse on our journey to heal what can't be erased is the necessary process of grieving our losses. We'll cover that next.

PERSONALIZE IT

THE POINT

The art of surrender is less about giving *up* than about giving *in* to a process of confrontation that will lead to the transformation of our lives from the inside out. Surrender requires truth. Surrender requires a transfer of our outer garments. And it requires tethering to the Vine, who is Christ.

THE PROMPT

What are your outer garments that need to be thrown at the feet of Jesus? Ungrieved losses? Unresolved disappointments? Regret? Insecurity? Victimhood? Today is your day to cease finding sufficiency and identity in your deficiencies.

THE POSTURE

What specific choices will you make to take responsibility for stewarding the life you have been given and to sever your ties with an identity defined by adversity? The burdens you've been carrying are far too heavy. Will you lay them down at Jesus's feet as we continue our journey together? He's calling you to move forward by His might!

THE PRAYER

Father, today I ask for the grace to surrender every true experience of pain, loss, and disappointment to You in exchange for the truth that will set me free. I throw my outer garments of self-protection at Your feet. Help me take courage and get up from the painful experiences of my past. You're calling me to Yourself, and I want to follow You wholeheartedly. I don't have what it takes to fix or heal myself. And I'm done trying to do it alone. Lead me today. In Jesus's name, amen.

SEVEN

NECESSARY GRIEVING

The reality is that you will grieve forever. You will not "get over" the loss of a loved one; you will learn to live with it. You will heal, and you will rebuild yourself around the loss you have suffered. You will be whole again, but you will never be the same. Nor should you be the same, nor would you want to.

—ELISABETH KÜBLER-ROSS and DAVID KESSLER,
On Grief and Grieving

For the first few months or so after my mom passed away, I barely spoke. Not only did I lack words, but I struggled to muster the energy to utter them even when they arrived. In fact, most of my interactions with people consisted of simple nods. During that same time, I didn't touch the stove either. It was once a place that represented my love, care, and devotion to my family but now triggered trauma. It didn't matter that much, I guess, because it's not like I had much of an appetite to begin with.

My body was often cold and my skin clammy. I would fall asleep crying and wake up with new tears rolling down my swollen, pale cheeks, even though I don't remember any significant emotion accompanying those tears. On second thought, maybe that was because I had only one continuous emotion: deep sadness. When I was awake throughout the day, I felt like I was observing life unfolding without actively participating in it, as if I were disconnected from my body and those around me. It was all white noise.

And though the sun still rose and set each day, though the traffic lights never ceased to change on cue, and despite the fact that dinner wasn't going to make itself, my life was monotone and hazy, blurry and undefined. No doubt the shock of my recent loss was running full tilt. It pervaded every corner of my being and every moment of every day. As autumn turned to winter and winter turned to spring in those first several months after Mom died, my "Groundhog Day" continued. Then months later came Mother's Day 2013, our first without her.

The year prior, I remember writing her a lengthy card that detailed how much I loved her, how she inspired me, how committed I was to her care, and how I looked forward to her healing—an unknown but long-anticipated day in the future when we could celebrate together and return to life as it should be. As you now know, that day never came. That Mother's Day, I rummaged through her nightstand and found the card tucked in a worn-out plastic bag. Slumping on the floor beside her bed, I read the words that I had written with such conviction and determination a year earlier. I whispered, "Happy Mother's Day, Mom," as a few tears dropped on the card, smudging the ink. I sat in silence for several more minutes. One of our dogs joined me and laid her head on my lap as if to say, *I miss her too.*

As I stood up, I couldn't have anticipated the torrent of emotion that suddenly crashed in on my heart. I collapsed on the neatly made bed where Mom once lay, sheets untouched in months. I screamed and then screamed louder. I shook uncontrollably as this hurricane of unfamiliar emotion overwhelmed me. Nearly seven months of whispers gave way to an eruption of pain that had been brewing beneath the surface all that time.

For two hours, alone in the house, I lay across her bed while my soul battled against the unanswered questions surrounding this defeat it had been dealt. It wasn't pretty, but it was necessary.

The place where she once slept and took her last breath was a hallowed space. Because she was cremated, there was no grave site. The room that was once her haven became her memorial ground and the meeting place for my soul. It was as if it had to happen there, perhaps for closure in some way. No doubt, I was living David's words from Psalm 6:6: "I am weary with my moaning;

—

every night I flood my bed with tears; I drench my couch with my weeping."

This is grief: unpredictable like a wild river, unbearable with its violent force, yet also subtle, numbing, and all-encompassing. Had my love for her, my commitment to her care for nearly twenty years, and my dashed expectations for her healing in this life amounted to the profundity and depth of grief I was experiencing? I believe so, and I think the same will be true for you in your own life. In fact, it has been said, "The pain of grief is just as much a part of life as the joy of love; it is, perhaps, the price we pay for love, the cost of commitment."[1]

Unavoidable Grief

Whether it's due to a loved one's death, a job loss, major or minor life changes, betrayal, or divorce, experiencing grief is inevitable and unavoidable. Anytime we undergo change in life, we experience a measure of loss. And loss must be grieved. One biblical scholar put language to this, and wrote, "There is no attempt in Scripture to whitewash the anguish of God's people when they undergo suffering. They argue with God, they complain to God, they weep before God. Theirs is not a faith that leads to dry-eyed stoicism, but a faith so robust it wrestles with God."[2]

As ubiquitous as the experience of grief is, however, its expression is as unique as one's fingerprint.[3] Moreover, when it comes to healing from life circumstances that can never be erased, we sometimes overlook the notion that grief is not only helpful but also indisputably necessary.

In the previous chapter, we talked about surrender through the approaches of truth telling, transferring the weight of our burdens (throwing off our outer garments), and tethering ourselves to the Vine anew. And in many ways, I believe grieving is a primary vehicle by which we initiate surrender in all three modes. Grieving requires us to face our pain head-on. Grieving is the process by which we release the weight of our sorrow and the devastation of our souls on the Lord in total honesty and vulnerability. And grieving shows us that we need to receive strength that is not our own, through community, in order to heal.

Facing our pain, revisiting loss, and exposing our wounds is a painful process. But I also believe that the broken soil of our hearts is where the Holy Spirit can do His most transformative work in us. Consequently, we must participate. We must allow this work to take place. *We must grieve,* for if we don't, we will eventually (even unintentionally) normalize life with intensified stored pain. And that stored pain affects our spirits, souls, and bodies. How? Well, it's like carrying a backpack full of heavy bricks with us each day— the weight of ungrieved losses and unresolved disappointments in our lives that, left unaddressed, give way to a spirit of unbelief.

And while we cannot control the specific process or length of our grieving, *until* we grieve, *until* we do the hard work of naming and facing our pain in the Lord's presence and with our community—meaning those who provide witness to our sorrow without tacking on the silver lining[4]—much of our emotional and physical energy is attached to the past and we remain stuck and traumatized in the cycle of pain we discussed in chapter 3. Grief work, therefore, is not simply human work; it is *healing* work.

Scripture is replete with verses about grief and loss, which tells us a couple of things. First, grief and loss are common to our human experience. But second, our Father is not unaware or distant from us in our pain. Was not Jesus Himself "a man of sorrows and acquainted with grief"?[5] Indeed, "He heals the brokenhearted and binds up their wounds."[6] I want to look at the stories of two people in the Scriptures that illuminate the posture of grief and also validate our shared experiences with it.

> Grief work is not simply human work; it is *healing* work.

HANNAH'S STORY

In 1 Samuel 1, we are introduced to Elkanah, a man who had two wives, Hannah and Peninnah. Peninnah had children, but Hannah had none. Not only was Hannah's barrenness met with cultural shame and the potential for ostracization,[7] but Peninnah provoked her to grief and irritation, exacerbating her pain to the point where Hannah would not eat. Elkanah responded to Hannah's distress by asking, "Why do you weep? And why do you not eat? And why is your heart sad? Am I not more to you than ten sons?"[8] Hannah then demonstrated a critical posture in relation to grief: We must not deny it or run away from it but instead face it with vulnerability and without reservation. Verses 9 and 10 read,

"After they had eaten and drunk in Shiloh, *Hannah rose.* Now Eli the priest was sitting on the seat beside the doorpost of the temple of the LORD. She was *deeply distressed* and prayed to the LORD *and wept bitterly.*"

Therein, we witness Hannah's unwillingness to hide or even internalize her pain. Expressing our sorrow unabashedly and entering the grief process help us eventually move forward in life without getting stuck in a moment or memory of what was. Often I tell people that grieving is like a bridge between two pieces of land. The bridge might be long, narrow, full of unexpected twists and turns, and unpleasant, but it is the necessary (and only) passageway to moving forward on our journey through life after loss.

> Expressing our sorrow unabashedly and entering the grief process help us eventually move forward in life without getting stuck in a moment or memory of what was.

The second key to effective grieving we see through Hannah's story is that in her pain, she moved *toward* the Lord, not away from Him. In fact, her prayers and petitions were so fervent and emotional that Eli, the priest, thought her stammering lips were the result of intoxication. But it was not so. Hannah told him, "I am a woman troubled in spirit. I have drunk neither wine nor strong drink, but I have been pouring out my soul before the LORD."[9]

As I shared in an earlier chapter, ungrieved loss and pain have a way of encouraging us to disconnect from the Vine and from our community of support and counsel, selling isolation as the safest place to live. But as we both know, isolation not only makes us vulnerable to believing lies about the trustworthy, careful attention of the Lord and of those who love us most in our time of pain and loss; it also severs our connection to our ultimate Source of Life and Hope, who is Christ. Allow me to revisit a principle I shared in chapter 3.

While nothing can separate us from the love of God, we essentially choose to separate ourselves from Him through isolation. In doing so, we become vulnerable to the ingrowth of a "root of bitterness" within our hearts that brings defilement.[10] Consequently, isolation sequesters us to a barren place within, where despair and the broken spirit thrive.

Hannah's story also teaches us the importance of coming to the Lord in truth and honesty, pouring out our hearts before Him with specificity in our cries and petitions. After Eli approached her thinking she was drunk, Hannah responded, "Do not regard your servant as a worthless woman, for all along I have been speaking out of my great anxiety and vexation."[11] Verses 17 and 18 continue, "Then Eli answered, 'Go in peace, and the God of Israel grant your petition that you have made to him.' And she said, 'Let your servant find favor in your eyes.' Then the woman went her way and ate, and her face was no longer sad."

> Moving through grief allows us to move forward in life.

Herein is the takeaway: Moving through grief allows us to move forward in life. But when we don't face our grief head-on and move *through* the grief process, we complicate matters and remain stuck in the particular season of life marked by loss. And that ungrieved loss and defeat (our defining moment when *it* happened) will determine how we live out each day both now and in the future. It will serve as the distorted lens through which we see ourselves and the world around us.

That's why Hannah's story is worth studying. She modeled for us a healthy example of moving through grief toward healing. But what I find interesting is that Hannah's circumstance did not change immediately, even after she grieved before the Lord and the priest assured her that the Lord heard her prayers. What *did* change was her countenance and the disposition of her soul—not to mention her appetite. Perhaps, then, the ultimate goal of mourning is to help us move beyond our initial reactions and cope with the loss in a healthy way.[12] Just like Job.

JOB'S STORY

Job's story, familiar to many of us, is another powerful narrative about grief and loss. Scripture says that Job was "blameless and upright, one who feared God and turned away from evil."[13] Prosperous and influential, this father of ten was living the good life until one day when utter chaos and devastation swooped down and destroyed his livestock, his servants, and his children. Nearly everything that held a place of value in his life was gone in an instant.

What happened next was a profound display of shock and anguish. In a state of distress and horror, Job ripped his robe, shaved his head, and dropped to his knees in worship as he cried out, "I came naked from my mother's womb, and I will be naked when I leave. The LORD gave me what I had, and the LORD has taken it away. Praise the name of the LORD!"[14]

Like Hannah, Job demonstrated that the nature of grief is not only primeval but also devastating, all-consuming, and even debilitating—and it must be met with honest, uninhibited lament. It *must*. Certainly, while the Lord is not the author of sickness, disease, or destruction in our lives, pain and heartache are inevitable in this world that awaits God's redemption and full restoration. And that pain must be acknowledged, felt, and grieved.

Let's continue in Job's story. After having lost his children, his servants, and thousands of livestock, Job was struck with painful sores from head to toe.[15] As Job sat in an ash heap, scraping himself with a piece of broken pottery in hopes of alleviating the pain, his wife was obviously exasperated and furious by the devastation imposed on her family's livelihood. She probed her husband, "Do you still hold fast your integrity? Curse God and die."[16] He responded, " 'You speak as one of the foolish women would speak. Shall we receive good from God, and shall we not receive evil?' In all this Job did not sin with his lips."[17]

Shortly thereafter, Job's friends caught wind of his losses and knew they needed to respond. There's much to learn from them, too, specifically about how (and how not) to interact with others in their times of grief. Let's take a look at what happened.

WALKING WITH OTHERS THROUGH GRIEF

Before Job's friends opened their mouths and caused more harm than good in his situation, they modeled a helpful posture when serving those we love in their times of loss. Job 2:11–13 says, "When Job's three friends heard of all this evil that had come upon him, they came each from his own place, Eliphaz the Temanite, Bildad the Shuhite, and Zophar the Naamathite. They made an appointment together to come to show him sympathy and comfort him. And when they saw him from a distance, they did not recognize him. And they raised their voices and wept, and they tore their robes and sprinkled dust on their heads toward heaven. And they sat with him on the ground seven days and seven nights, and *no one spoke a word to him,* for they saw that his suffering was very great."

> When we're mourning, we need presence, not platitudes.

When we're mourning, we need presence, not platitudes. I'll never forget some of the strange things people said to me and my family after Mom went to be with the Lord. Three weeks after she passed, someone approached me out in public, acting as if he were excited to deliver some fresh advice. "Well, you know, Chris," he said as he leaned in, "God moves in mysterious ways."

Puzzled, annoyed, and still in a haze of shock, I quietly replied, "God didn't say that. Bono said that."

Squinting his eyes and cocking his head like a golden retriever who heard "treat," he probed, "*Who?*"

"Bono, the lead singer of the band U2. That was *his* line, not God's," I bluntly clarified as I turned around and walked away.

Then there was the mixtape featuring these hot takes: "God must have needed her," "We still won," and "Everything works out for good."

Topping the charts about a month later, another man approached me and asked, "Are you all better now? It's been a couple of months, right?"

Sarcasm and disdain ran through my mind. *You know, come to think of it, between losing my mom after her eighteen-year battle with cancer and this paper cut from yesterday, I am all better.*

You've probably heard other renditions of insensitive questions and clichés in your own situation. I don't know about you, but I hated those moments, and I hated their words. I braced myself for them, in fact. Sadly, too many came my way. But I doubt that anyone with half a heart planned for malice or insensitivity in their response to my grief.

> When people are hurting, they don't need explanations. They need *us*. Show up and shut up.

So why does it happen? And why do we do it to others? I think it's because we're incredibly uncomfortable with situations as severe as death and we simply don't know what to say. Imagine falling out of a boat into choppy waters at sea and struggling to stay afloat as wave after wave pummeled you. In that moment, you wouldn't need anyone to coach you through understanding the process that led to your falling overboard, right? You'd just need someone to pull you out of the water. And thus, my point: When people are hurting, they don't need explanations. They need *us*. Show up and shut up. When Lazarus died, Jesus, the *only* one who could change the situation in an instant, didn't preach a sermon about how all things work together for good. He wept. I think we should take His cue and do the same.

GRIEF CHANGES US

Grief changes us . . . *all* of us. As we see through the entirety of Job's story, the process of grieving will eventually lead to the healing of our hearts, not because time alone heals—*it doesn't*—but because a tender heart, broken and laid bare before Jesus's feet, will be embraced and met with the supernatural comfort of a loving Father. Even with all our doubts, questions, and feelings of anger and betrayal, in His time God will restore what appears to be broken and hopeless. But absent of this necessary course of mourning, we disconnect and separate ourselves from Him. Just as it did with Job's wife, such separation produces a hardened heart and bitterness.

Through my own and others' journeys of bereavement, I've discovered that we all end up with scars. And those scars tell a story. But the question is, What story will *your* scars tell? One of loss *with* restoration because you have grieved wholeheartedly? Or one of bitterness like those "who have no hope"?[18]

My point is that in the metanarrative of healing what can never be erased in our lives, grieving is a necessary and prominent player. We must engage with it if we want to heal. The Lord comforts all who mourn, but I do not believe we will ever receive the fullness of comfort He offers and readily provides until we willingly and vulnerably come into His presence with our fractured hearts.

THE POSTURE AND PATH OF GRIEF

Having investigated Hannah's and Job's stories of grief and mourning, I want to run a thread through the two narratives to paint an even clearer picture of the dynamics of this delicate, crucial process. Hannah and Job, as well as David, Jesus, and others in Scripture, demonstrate the importance of approaching grief with the posture of truth and vulnerability. Once again, I turn to the wisdom of my friend Curt Thompson to expound on this thought. He wrote, "Genuine, healthy grieving is a necessary part of the experience of loss. But when grief is not addressed openly and vulnerably, it can keep us from entering new relationships—stuck in isolation, cut off from others."[19]

And when we remain stuck in isolation, unwilling to do the hard, critical work of grieving our losses, we inevitably step off the tracks while the train called "life" is still moving forward. Sadly, this is the story of too many people, their lives derailed because of ungrieved losses and unresolved disappointments. The arduous process of grieving is therefore the necessary bridge from unforgettable pain and loss to transformation and wholeness. Grief is not something we just "get over," because, as I stated earlier, time alone will not heal our broken hearts. Instead, grieving is a process we move through—a winding and uneven path our souls tread upon. Through our grieving, we are changed from the inside out by the power of the Holy Spirit and in our community of care and support.

Thankfully, we have various tools and strategies available to help put us back on track as we continue to move forward in life after loss. We've discussed several in this chapter alone. But in addition to these strategies, we have been given a helpful framework for putting language to the experiences within the grief process itself. Such was the work of renowned psychiatrist Elisabeth Kübler-Ross.

In 1969, Elisabeth Kübler-Ross plotted out the five stages of dying in her landmark book *On Death and Dying*. Her protégé, David Kessler, later partnered with her to adapt and better align the five stages with the experiences of those who were not dying but grieving. Their work led them to document the following five stages of grief:

Denial: shock and disbelief that the loss has occurred
Anger: that someone we love is no longer here
Bargaining: all the what-ifs and regrets
Depression: sadness for the loss
Acceptance: acknowledging the reality of the loss[20]

Of great importance, as Kessler pointed out in his book *Finding Meaning,* "the five stages were never intended to be prescriptive,"[21] as if we could compartmentalize the grief process and its intense emotions in a tidy conveyor belt–like procedure. Instead, as Kessler wrote, these stages "describe only a general process. Each person grieves in his or her own unique way. Nonetheless, the grieving process does tend to unfold in similar stages to what we described, and most people who have gone through it will recognize them."[22]

I want to point out that the fifth stage, acceptance, does not infer that we will ever be okay with the loss or even that the grief process is over—not in the slightest! Instead, as Kessler explained, acceptance simply means that we have acknowledged the finality and permanence of the loss.[23]

So, the posture of the grief process requires openness, honesty, and vulnerability in the presence of the Lord and our community, and the *path* of grief unfolds like a rocky, uneven terrain. In light of this, I'd like to propose that the *reach* of grief extends to the depths of our souls, our physiology, and our human spirits.

THE REACH OF GRIEF

Think about your own grief. What did it feel like? How did it affect your outlook on (and interactions with) everyday life? In the height of my grief, I felt overwhelmed by an unrelenting weight and inescapable pressure from both outside and inside so that trying to focus or accomplish much in life was both strenuous and exhausting. Scripture says that the Lord will never leave me or forsake me,[24] but why, then, did it feel like I had been abandoned and left for dead when I needed Him the most? Kessler gave us a clue when he wrote that "grief grabs your heart and doesn't seem to let go."[25] *That's* why. Grief is so invasive that it steers our focus and steals our energy. But without mourning, we won't move through the grief. Instead, we will remain stuck and consumed in our past.

Another medical researcher painted a brilliant picture of grief. She said, "The experience of being swept by the river is emblematic to me of losing a loved one through death. The overwhelming sensation of being at a complete loss, flooded with sorrow, incapacitated with aching. Consciously breathing, but not sensing any oxygen."[26] Can you relate? I believe these metaphors point to grief's systemic effects on us—in other words, the *reach* of grief. Grief manifests itself not only in depression, anxiety, sadness, numbness, and myriad other emotions but also in physiological changes that occur in our bodies due to the biochemical effects of those emotions. Symptoms such as sleeplessness, memory loss, fatigue, appetite loss, headaches, muscle tension, irritability, and digestive troubles are common.[27]

But the experience of grief can also affect us spiritually, distorting our perception of the Lord's nearness and care for us in times of pain and loss, as if we were wearing blurry eyeglasses. As a result, many of us distrust and doubt the very assurances we read in the Word.

Remember David, who cried to the Lord in Psalm 13:1–2, "How long, O Lord? Will you forget me forever? How long will you hide your face from me? How long must I take counsel in my soul and have sorrow in my heart all the day? How long shall my enemy be exalted over me?" And again, in Psalm 22:1–2, he wrote, "My God, my God, why have you forsaken me? Why are you so far from saving me, from the words of my groaning? O my God, I cry by day, but you do not answer, and by night, but I find no rest." Though David's experiences were painful and his feelings were real, had the Lord actually forsaken him? Had He forgotten him? And does He abandon *us*? Certainly not. But in times of grief and loss, it feels that way, doesn't it?

In life, it's easy to lose perspective of the truth when we're overwhelmed by the blistering facts staring us in the face, isn't it? You know what I'm talking about: the divorce papers on the table, the empty chair at Thanksgiving dinner, the loved one's lifeless body in the casket, the eviction notice tacked to the front door, or the phone call from the doctor with a devastating medical diagnosis. These are the precise moments in which mourning and lament are not only helpful but also critical.

Through our vulnerability and sorrow, as our hearts remain tender before Him, God's transformative power does its finest work of true healing that leads to wholeness. This is another key point I want you to understand. Tender hearts that are yielded in trust to the Father through every victory *and* every loss can receive the fullness of all that He has for us in this life. Why? Because the condition of our hearts determines the course of our lives.[28] And through the *transformation* of our hearts, we will experience a measure of restoration not fathomable (or attainable) by the rational mind. This is the great exchange the Father promised us: comfort for our mourning; beauty for our ashes; the oil of gladness instead of our mourning; and the garment of praise instead of our faint, broken spirits.[29] Some would argue that this soul exchange is impossible, a pipe dream even. But because I've seen this supernatural mystery unfold in my own life, I want your faith to be strengthened by my experience and convictions on the matter.

About a year after my mom had passed and shortly after my MS diagnosis—right in the middle of personal chaos where I could barely see straight—my pastor reminded me that these storms would sharpen the call of God on my life. Now to clarify, in no way was he insinuating that cancer or MS was the authorship of the Lord. Banish the thought! Instead, I believe he meant that there was no limit to the Lord's ability to redeem these devastating circumstances for His purposes and thus restore me to wholeness. And that brushstroke of redemption—how the Lord works *all things* together for our good[30]—is a great mystery to all of us who entrust our lives to Him.

But the key to experiencing it is baring our whole hearts before the Lord without reservation. I believe what the Scriptures say in

Ephesians 3:20–21: "To him who is able to do far more abundantly than all that we ask or think, *according to the power at work within us,* to him be glory in the church and in Christ Jesus throughout all generations, forever and ever. Amen." Yet look at the condition: it's according to the dynamic, miraculous, transformative power of His Spirit that works in us. For His power to work in us, we must partner with Him through yielded hearts that are unwilling to be defined by the defeat of broken spirits.

THE CONSEQUENCES OF AVOIDING THE GRIEF PROCESS

Having said that, I'm still curious about why many of us either avoid or step timidly into the grief process, even though we know that loss in life is inevitable and that facing our pain is necessary for healing. I think the answer is that we don't like the feeling of powerlessness.

"The element of powerlessness," Brené Brown wrote, "is what makes anguish traumatic. We are unable to change, reverse, or negotiate what has happened. And even in those situations where we can temporarily reroute anguish with to-do lists and tasks, it finds its way back to us."[31]

We don't like the feeling of losing control, which is exactly what we must do when we grieve—we must give up control of the process and its timing, of outcomes, and of others' reactions. So, in an effort to feign control, we get busy. We fill our hearts, minds, and schedules with the white noise of meetings, overcommitment, Netflix, and Instagram. Add to that, if we don't like feeling out of control and already feel as though our hands are tied behind our backs because of past trauma and loss, why would we voluntarily revisit the same spaces of our hearts that once met us with excruciating pain and anguish? Why would we want to open our soul wounds afresh?

> In an effort to feign control, we get busy.

But avoiding issues doesn't make them go away; it actually

makes them more permanent. Sadly, when we choose to avoid any semblance of the past as well as the people, places, conversations, and experiences that remind us of what we lost, we cause more complicated and exacerbated pain long-term. I totally understand if that describes you right now. However, the consequences of avoiding the grief process are even more devastating over time, because grief that becomes complicated hampers our ability to cope with even the normal demands of everyday life.

This is yet another key I want you to apprehend regarding the necessity of grieving our losses. Avoiding grief, as painful as it is, does not allow us to bypass the effects of grief.

COMPLICATED GRIEF

Complicated grief, I believe, consumes us and redefines us, but not in a way that points to healing and transformation. Instead, it defines us by defeat and despair. "A person with complicated grief feels intense emotional pain. . . . A future without their loved one seems forever dismal and unappealing," an article from the Center for Prolonged Grief explains. "Grief dominates their thoughts and feelings with no respite in sight. . . . Life can seem purposeless, like nothing seems to matter without their loved one."[32]

Instead of avoiding, numbing, or ignoring these pain-filled places of our hearts—where we keep our greatest unanswered questions—what would happen if we acknowledged, made space for, and submitted them to the mighty hand of the Lord (with our counselor's assistance), where He and *only* He can exchange our ashes for beauty? This is what finding meaning through loss is all about.

FINDING MEANING AND EMBRACING MYSTERY

How would you respond if I told you that you could find meaning through every loss you've endured? Not the answer to *why* it happened. Not an opportunity to close the loop of cognitive dissonance or suddenly be okay with the loss either. But an opportunity to build a memorial called "meaning," a reflection of the love you have for that which you've lost.[33] And meaning, according to David Kessler, is the sixth stage of grief.[34] Finding meaning won't give you an answer for why you lost your loved one . . . or your job . . . or your hope. Rather, it will continue to allow the hand of your Creator, who happens to be your Father, to write your life's story. And it will help you recognize that while the soul blows of grief will soften over time, grief in this fallen world will never completely end.[35]

Maybe that's why I'm realizing all over again, even as I write these words, that finding meaning after loss requires us to do something rather foreign to our souls and off-putting to our penchants toward platitudes and pat answers when crises crash on our hearts. We have to learn how to embrace mystery.

Why wasn't my mom healed on this side of eternity? I don't know. Why did my body seem to betray me in the height of my pain and unmask an autoimmune disease? I don't know. Why did *it* happen to you? I don't know. But honestly, I believe "I don't know" is the correct answer. A cookie-cutter answer won't work because of the discomfort we feel when sitting in a state of pain. "I don't know" leaves us with *mystery*. Again, finding meaning *requires us* to embrace mystery. I was reminded of this through the words of a pastor walking through grief himself. He wrote, "Our trust in God is seldom seen in what we understand. Our trust is often proven and established by what we do with mystery. This is one of the most neglected areas of the faith—treasuring mystery."[36] I believe he's correct.

Even though you will never move on from your loss, it is possible for you to move forward. So, will you drop your self-protection and your proclivity toward isolation in the presence of the Lord today? I know you might be jaded and cynical about hope after heartbreak. I totally get it. I was there ten years ago. But He's eager to heal and transform you if you'll allow Him to do so. Will it hurt? Yes, it will, my friend. And will you have to re-expose wounds that have scabbed over but not necessarily healed properly? Yes to that too. But just as I said in the last chapter, when your wounds meet the hands of the Wounded Healer, His stripes not only heal but also make the broken whole.

> Healing what can never be erased isn't about forgetting your past. It's about throwing off every weight that holds you down and living the overcoming life to which you were called by a careful, loving Father.

Healing what can never be erased isn't about forgetting your past or living some superficial life of denial. It's about throwing off every weight that holds you down and living the overcoming life to which you were called by a careful, loving Father. Today might be your first day to take your first step toward wholeness. But I'm right here to walk alongside you. Transformation is nigh, my friend. Believe me.

PERSONALIZE IT

THE POINT

Because grief is an unavoidable experience for all of us, entering the grief process is a necessary trek that helps us eventually move forward in life.

THE PROMPT

How has grief affected your soul, your physiology, and even your spirit?

THE POSTURE

Grief is unpredictable like a wild river, unbearable with its violent force yet subtle, numbing, and all-encompassing. Therefore, we must not deny or run away from our grief but face it with vulnerability and without reservation. Feel it, journal it, cry through it, sleep through it, and continue to pour your whole heart out to the Lord. The great paradox is that you will heal as you mourn. You never have to move on from your losses, but because you're reading a book about healing what you can't erase, I'm confident you want to move forward.

THE PRAYER

Lord, I know that the consequences of avoiding the grief process are even more devastating over time, because grief that becomes complicated hampers my ability to cope with even the normal demands of everyday life. Therefore, I ask for Your help and invite You into my grief process. Teach me how to pour out my heart to You, especially when I'm afraid to do so. You promise to comfort all who mourn. And right now, that's me. Here's my broken, bereaved heart. I receive the peace and comfort of the Holy Spirit now in the strong name of Jesus. Amen.

EIGHT

THE PATHWAY TO PEACE

> Peace I leave with you; my peace I give to you. Not as the
> world gives do I give to you. Let not your hearts be
> troubled, neither let them be afraid.
>
> —JESUS CHRIST, John 14:27

Unaddressed pain, unresolved disappointment, anxious and fore-boding thoughts, and even anticipatory grief are like a vacuum. They suck our energy, our focus, and, most specifically, our courage. Because of the accumulation of circumstances in my life, I was so afraid of ever experiencing that level of unrelenting pain again. So, I tried my best to put a stranglehold on my life and my routine so that nothing would happen without my consent. From the inside out, it made sense. But from the outside in, it was *crazy*—and I don't mean to use that word lightly. The obsessive-compulsive drive to avoid pain provoked me to steer clear of anything that was reminiscent of the past: certain roads, music, foods, and even television shows.

And while I understand the triggers of trauma, I was insulating and self-protecting my heart so much that I created a new normal that was anything but. The compulsion waged war on my mental and emotional health to the extent that I lost sight of how to live a normal life. Some days I wasn't sure I even wanted to live. My efforts were aimed not only at avoiding traumatic triggers but also, I now realize, at trying to stop the hemorrhaging within my soul. It seemed as if the more I grieved, the more layers of buried pain came to the surface. When the bleeding would stop, I did not know. All I knew was that I wanted some peace.

Yet the harder I fought for peace by eliminating potential triggers, reducing my life to what I thought I could control, and avoiding anything that could potentially be ripped from me, the further peace seemed to drift away from me. Worse, my neurotic drive for predictability and stability only ramped up the very fear and anxiety I was trying to rid from my life. The cycle felt like a cruel joke, honestly. As it turned out, though, I was the one perpetuating the madness through the unbridled climate of internal chaos and my subsequent attempts at self-preservation. Can you relate? Especially after an elongated period of stress in life, we want the chaos to stop; we want the storm clouds to part, right? And that's how we like to define peace too: "an absence of conflict." In his song "Imagine," John Lennon shared this sentiment about peace, positioning it as a nebulous absence of anything "to kill or die for." It's what he aimed for but could never attain. Peace, according to Lennon, is a world without heaven. No hell either. No possessions to call your own. *Nothing.* He calls *that* "peace."[1]

But what if our expectations of what peace looks like are keeping us from actually experiencing it? *Real* peace is not a soul state absent of conflict; it is one in which the omnipotent presence of the Prince of Peace indwells every circumstance and trial. It is a kingdom commodity as strong as a military force standing watch over our hearts and minds without relenting. This peace is a fruit borne by the Holy Spirit in those whom Jesus, the Vine, called "branches." Its seed is mighty, containing the genetic code of wholeness. Its root system is deep, having been planted beside rivers of living water. And *this* peace is Jesus's very own, which He freely confers on us.[2]

In chapter 3, we learned about interrupting and escaping the cycle of pain, the environment in which the broken spirit thrives. Chapter 6 presented the way out: surrender through telling the truth, transferring our burdens, and tethering ourselves to the

Vine. And in chapter 7, we learned why grieving our losses is a necessary factor in the process of surrender. This chapter is aimed at receiving and walking in peace, which results from a life that has been surrendered to and is abiding in Christ.

I want to frame a couple of scriptures from the outset to establish a foundation on which to build our discussion. Isaiah 26:3–4 says,

> You keep him in perfect peace
>   whose mind is stayed on you,
>   because he trusts in you.
> Trust in the LORD forever,
>   for the LORD GOD is an everlasting rock.

When our minds are "stayed" on Him, our mindsets—our total way of looking at things—are steady and undeviating,[3] fixed on the Lord, and the result is perfect peace. In the Old Testament, the word for "peace" is the Hebrew word *shâlôm,* from the root word *shâlam,* which means "to be safe, sound, healthy, perfect, complete" and "signifies a sense of well-being and harmony both within and without." It involves "completeness, wholeness, peace, health, welfare, safety, soundness, tranquility, prosperity, fullness, rest, harmony; the absence of agitation or discord, a state of calm without anxiety or stress."[4] In other words, perfect peace, as prescribed by Scripture, offers holistic health to our innermost beings: our spirits and souls. This will affect our physical health too.

Looking into the New Testament, in John 14:27, Jesus said to His disciples, "Peace I leave with you; My [own] peace I now give and bequeath to you. Not as the world gives do I give to you. Do not let your hearts be troubled, neither let them be afraid. [Stop allowing yourselves to be agitated and disturbed; and do not permit yourselves to be fearful and intimidated and cowardly and unsettled]" (AMPC). The Greek word for "peace" used here is *eirēnē,* which, much like the Hebrew *shâlôm,* conveys a sense of well-being and inner rest.[5] Moreover, Jesus's statement that he would "leave" His peace with His disciples is akin to a legacy given by one departing.[6] And this legacy of peace is ours in Christ just the same!

With all this in mind, I'd like to propose the following equation:

A Fixed Focus + Well-Established Trust =
Perfect Peace (Wholeness)

Now, there's a chance you just rolled your eyes at seeing "well-established trust" in that equation. After all, how presumptuous of me to tell you that you need to rekindle the very thing that was shattered into a million pieces after *it* happened. And how insensitive of me to neatly package up your pain and send you on your way without giving you a moment to gain your bearings. Stay with me. Trust takes way more time to build (or rebuild) than the mere moment in which it can be destroyed. I'm not ignorant of that. So, my thesis—my extended arm to you—isn't a flimsy platitude. I do believe it is the right equation, but as you'll soon learn, our approach back to trust will take on a new form because it has a different target than where many of us previously aimed.

Exhale. Are we good? Let's continue. I'll unpack the equation for you now.

If I *fix my focus* without *trusting* in the power, wisdom, and goodness of the Lord, I have mere religion. For example, I can be devoted to the steadfast tradition of faith and even know what the Bible says without my heart or my life being actively engaged with (and validating) my professed devotion.[7] Is my focus fixed? Sure, in a way. But because it isn't met with demonstrable abiding trust in the Lord as a preeminent, undergirding value of my life, I have what Paul describes as the appearance of godliness without its power.[8] About this, one scholar commented, "For Paul, religion without God's power transforming the heart was useless."[9]

On the other hand, the fabric of my trust must be shaped by the principles of the Word and founded on the Lord's character expressed by His self-revelation through Scripture. If it's shaped by my limited perspective and expectations instead, I'm setting myself up for potential disappointment (let alone a life of emotional instability and spiritual immaturity) anytime adversity comes my way. In other words, crisis and adversity have a way of revealing the substance of our trust.

Think about your own life. Is the foundation of your trust framed by your own expectations? By the certainty of an outcome? By your own insight, ability, or understanding? Or is your trust anchored by your fixed focus on the One who said that *no matter what* you encounter in life, He will never leave you or forsake you?[10] And that all things work together for good for those who love God and are called according to His purpose?[11] Without a doubt, a fixed focus and well-established trust work hand in hand. This is further evidence of why Solomon admonished us to "trust in, and be confident in the Lord with all your heart and mind and do not rely on your own insight or understanding."[12]

David captured the same principle in Psalm 16:8 when he wrote, "I have set the LORD always before me; because he is at my right hand, I shall not be shaken." The point is that whatever we focus on flourishes. And whatever we magnify in our hearts gets magnified in how we live out each day. Don't miss this. The issue isn't whether or not we will fix our focus at all but what we focus on—that is, the object of our focus. Moreover, when we lack focus *and* trust, we're essentially living as people who are double-minded and unstable (unreliable and uncertain) in all our ways.[13]

This is why I want to fortify the foundational principles of focus and trust from the Scriptures. But first, by presenting the equation above, in no way am I inferring that peace is something we achieve through our own efforts. Peace is not a token we pull from a slot machine called "God." Certainly, we make choices and establish priorities in life to position ourselves to walk in peace, but peace is not achieved; it is received. Likewise, peace is the result not of striving but of surrender. Therefore, this equation must not be approached and outworked as a life hack, but instead, understood as the fruit of our abiding on the Vine—a posture I failed to maintain a short time ago.

A FIXED FOCUS

A couple of months ago, I awoke with an unusual level of exhaustion. It was soul deep, even though I couldn't pinpoint its origin. And though the fatigue manifested in my physical body, it crashed in on my emotions, too, in a very surprising way. I was irritable but not angry, and a few sleepless nights only made matters worse. However, I knew one more inconvenience or small defeat would most likely uncork a flood of tears that felt as trapped as the backed-up pipe I had just cleared underneath my kitchen sink. Candidly, I think I was actually hoping for that "one more thing" just to get those tears unstuck. Typically in these situations, I'm pretty good at naming my emotions, but for one reason or another, this time around I struggled to put language to the state of my soul. Then, while reading early one morning, I came across a quote by Father Ronald Rolheiser from his broader teaching on the various factors in life that steal our awareness of God's presence. Three sentences within the narrative completely arrested my attention:

> You are inside yourself, torn by your pain, endlessly reviewing past and future conversations, possibilities, and fantasies. . . . You are locked in an inner world whose obsessive reality absorbs all your awareness. . . . Your reality has been reduced to the size, shape, and color of your own inner world.[14]

Bullseye. Rolheiser's words, in almost prophetic fashion, gave clear expression to the underlying issues of my heart. It was a Spirit-led ambush in the best possible way, and the tears that had been painfully stuck flowed freely. *My* world had been reduced to the size, shape, and color of my own inner world—which was being steered by the chaos of circumstances far outside my control. The overwhelm felt all-consuming. But being a couple of days removed from the intensity of my circumstances, I realized that I had lost perspective, which stole my focus, which unhooked me from peace. My slow drift off the Vine was not intentional, of course, but slow and steady, by way of one unsurrendered burden at a time. And as a result, I was exhausted.

It goes without saying that adversity hurts, especially when it attacks like an ambush in the night. Times of shaking come to all of us. But there's great strength to be had when our focus is fixed, especially *in* the shaking. Psalm 16:8 is my life verse, and it speaks about the power of a fixed focus. Have a look at it in a few different translations:

I have *set* the LORD always before me;
    because he is at my right hand, *I shall not be shaken.* (ESV)

I have *set* the Lord continually before me; because He is at my right hand, *I shall not be moved.* (AMPC)

I *keep my eyes* always on the LORD.
    With him at my right hand, *I will not be shaken.* (NIV)

I *constantly trust* in the LORD;
because he is at my right hand, *I will not be shaken.* (NET)

I *know* the LORD is always with me.
    I will not be shaken, for he is right beside me. (NLT)

What's the common denominator? The *strength* to be had *by a fixed focus.* Now, does that mean that a fixed focus allows us to circumvent hard times? Obviously not. But the promise of the Word is that when our focus is fixed, *we* will not be shaken or upended when everything else around us is being shaken. Hence, my unsettledness—my lack of peace—stemmed from focus that had drifted away from the only One who is unshakable to everything that was being shaken around me.

Back to the equation. Though I trusted the Lord, my lack of focus hindered me from experiencing the peace that was readily available. And the same will be true for you too. Look again at

Jesus's words from the second half of John 14:27 in the Amplified Bible Classic Edition: "Do not let your hearts be troubled, neither let them be afraid. [*Stop allowing yourselves* to be agitated and disturbed; and *do not permit yourselves* to be fearful and intimidated and cowardly and unsettled]."

Could it be that agitation and intimidation come to us most easily (and are exacerbated) when we lose our focus? When the storms on the outside get on the inside? I'd like to think so.

That was me last week, to be honest. Approaching a routine doctor appointment and anticipating biopsy results, I was pummeled by an onslaught of irrational fear and anxiety. It came on me suddenly and surprisingly too. And as a result, writing this chapter has been a significant challenge—not because I don't believe these truths but because my focus had shifted away from the Prince of Peace who promised to never leave me or forsake me. If you think I'm totally free from this stuff just because I'm on this side of the page, think again.

Psalm 68:19 says, "Blessed be the Lord, Who bears our burdens and carries us day by day, even the God Who is our salvation!" (AMPC). I'm so thankful for that promise. He did exactly that. And every day last week on my four-mile walk through the neighborhood, I took the opportunity to refocus and strengthen myself in the Lord. Now, here we are, a full week after the appointment, and I just received a good report a few moments ago. *Exhale.* How's that for a case study on the power of a fixed focus? *Whatever* we focus on flourishes, and for me last week, it was anxiety and intimidation.

Back to Jesus's words, "Do not let your hearts be troubled." I find it interesting that He makes this bold, authoritative statement about receiving His very own peace only nine verses before He says, "I am the vine; you are the branches. Whoever abides in me and I in him, he it is that bears much fruit, for apart from me you can do nothing."[15] What's the point? Our ability to remain in peace is in equal proportion to our commitment to remain *in Him.* And when we remain in Him, one of those fruits of abiding is indeed peace.

In Colossians 3:15, the apostle Paul presents another valuable perspective about peace: It acts as an umpire and arbiter of questions and concerns that arise in our minds. I want you to see this verse in the Amplified Bible Classic Edition, specifically. Here's what he wrote: "Let the peace (soul harmony which comes) from Christ rule (act as umpire continually) in your hearts [deciding and *settling with finality all questions that arise in your minds,* in that peaceful state] to which as [members of Christ's] one body you were also called [to live]. And be thankful (appreciative), [giving praise to God always]." While the context of Colossians chapter 3 is about the perfect bond of love and the unity of the body of Christ, the broader principle is valuable for our application here. In realigning our thoughts to truth in Christ, we will reanchor our hearts in trust. And when peace is an umpire, deciding on the questions that arise in our minds, a fixed focus will allow us to discern truth from the false more expediently.

TRUE VS. TRUTH

A twentieth-century theologian wrote, "The way to right action is to appoint Jesus Christ as the arbiter between the conflicting emotions in our hearts; and if we accept his decisions, we cannot go wrong."[16] This is an important principle to understand because what's *true* to us isn't always *truth.* As I wrote in an earlier chapter, until our "true" is submitted to the Way, the Truth, and the Life Himself, we will continue to behave as "mere humans"[17] and lack the maturity and transformation to interact with the world in an effective way.

This is partly why I am so moved with compassion for anyone deluded into looking to oneself as the sole locus of guidance and authority for a meaningful life. Pardon my bluntness, but it's utter nonsense. Not one person trapped in that motivation is living freely in their true identity; instead, they're living in the self-supporting, self-preserving identity of an orphan. If peace is our desire, Christ must be our aim and anchor.

WELL-FOUNDED TRUST

Perfect peace is the summation of not only a fixed and undeterred focus but also a well-founded trust in the Lord. In Philippians 4:5–9, Paul wrote:

> The Lord is at hand; do not be anxious about anything, but in everything by prayer and supplication with thanksgiving let your requests be made known to God. And the peace of God, which surpasses all understanding, will guard your hearts and your minds in Christ Jesus.
>
> Finally, brothers, whatever is true, whatever is honorable, whatever is just, whatever is pure, whatever is lovely, whatever is commendable, if there is any excellence, if there is anything worthy of praise, think about these things. What you have learned and received and heard and seen in me—practice these things, and the God of peace will be with you.

For the Philippians to whom Paul wrote, worrying was a way of life. In addition to their apprehension about normal, everyday life, the threat of persecution for being a Christian triggered significant anxiety and motivated them to take life into their own hands.[18] Yet Paul's response was "Do not be anxious about anything." That's the precedent. It's a perspective shift for life, founded on trust and carried out through prayer.

Jesus's solution to our anxiety was for us to receive His peace by abiding in Him. Through that abiding, our focus becomes fixed and our trust established, empowering us to stop allowing ourselves to be agitated and disturbed.[19] Abiding infers trust. And in similar fashion, Paul gave this solution: "By prayer and supplication *with thanksgiving* let your requests be made known to God."[20] But why prayer *with* thanksgiving? Only when our hearts are assured that the Lord is working all things together for our good (there's the trust factor!) will we feel the gratitude that believing prayer requires.[21]

Then, in verse 7, Paul says that the peace that surpasses (transcends) all understanding will guard our whole inner beings like a military operative, ready to defend and protect without flinching. And as awesome as that promise is, the challenge is that too many of us trust in and lean on our own insight and understanding to the point that we have unknowingly chosen where to level off in our faith journeys. Sadly, as a result, we forfeit a supernatural experience of peace that is beyond the limitations of our understanding.

In other words, I've heard it said that we'll receive the peace that passes understanding only when we give up our right to understand.[22] No amount of human intellect or reason can produce this peace. William Barclay wrote, "It can never be of man's contriving; it is only of God's giving."[23]

Receiving the peace that passes our understanding also infers that we must learn how to live with mystery in our journeys of faith, especially in times of great loss. As we discussed in chapter 7, the answer to *why* might appear to be comforting at first glance, but it won't change the situation. After loss or disappointment, what we need is not an answer for why something did or did not happen but the supernatural peace of God, the comfort promised to all who mourn, and the healing of our broken hearts.

This is exactly why we are talking about peace *after* exploring the dynamics of grief—because healthy mourning leads us to experience peace with hope, while the absence of healthy mourning leads us toward separation, isolation, and unbelief. Hence, trusting in the Lord, especially when we can't yet ascribe meaning to our pain and loss, is a critical posture to learn and embody. To that end, I want to continue to reinforce the principle that our trust is not in the certainty of an outcome. Instead, well-founded trust rests in the character and nature of our mighty God who neither lies[24] nor changes.[25]

Taking the matter a step further, Solomon said, "Trust in the Lord with all your heart, and do not lean on your own understanding. In all your ways acknowledge him, and he will make straight your paths. Be not wise in your own eyes; fear the Lord, and turn away from evil. It will be healing to your flesh and refreshment to your bones."[26] Not only does unshakable trust in the Lord establish the peace that passes understanding, but anchoring ourselves on this wisdom produces health and wholeness in our bodies. That is stunning!

Moreover, trusting in and leaning on the Lord present an invitation to "taste and see that the LORD is good!"[27] Interestingly, when I read those verses in Proverbs again this week, the phrase "lean on" hit me in a fresh way. To lean on anything implies that weight is being transferred from one object to another. This is the essence of trust—and perhaps is a primary reason why so few people experience anything more than circumstantial peace in life. We unnecessarily carry our burdens ourselves because we don't trust people. And if we're honest, we probably even struggle to fully trust the Lord. Let's get under the hood and take a deeper look at some of the motivating reasons.

UNLOADING OUR BURDENS AND RELEARNING TRUST

If we've established that peace is the fruit of a surrendered life, one that is abiding on the Vine where focus is fixed and trust is established, the *absence* of peace clues us in to a few probable causes: disconnection from the Vine (independence and separateness), distraction from the Lord's instructions and promises found in Scripture, and hesitation to trust—seen in our tentativeness to lean on the Lord with the full weight of *every* burden, doubt, and fear in our hearts, even fear that brings torment. It has to start there!

Again, the thoroughness of our leaning is measured by the extent to which we willingly surrender and offload the weight of every burden we are bearing, including these:

- unresolved disappointments
- ungrieved losses
- fresh losses
- financial troubles

- health issues
- insecurities
- offenses and unforgiveness
- fears
- sin
- dreams and plans
- relationships
- languish in our souls

All those experiences are cumbersome. So why do we intentionally carry more in our souls than we ought? Well, as I said, I think many of us struggle to trust not only other people but also the steadfast character of the Lord—especially when what we see and feel with our natural senses overshadows our confidence in the abiding presence of the Comforter within us. His presence never leaves us. He *never* forsakes us. He *is* the same "yesterday and today and forever."[28] But in the heat of current painful circumstances and the unhealed memories of past disappointments, our *perception* of His presence is often compromised. We lose sight of truth that brings freedom, and thus our self-protective drive for control clamors, "Trust only yourself. Go at it alone." So, we do. We hide in shame. We disconnect and isolate. We think we know what's best for survival, but sadly, the end of that road is death.[29]

Listen, I get it. After people and life have let us down, trusting anyone or anything outside ourselves for life's defining moments is a real chore, isn't it? Trust indeed "requires a track record."[30] But a lack of trust keeps us from offloading these burdens and ultimately from stewarding this life in which God has called us to maturity as "more than conquerors"—those who not only receive His perfect peace but also are transformed and empowered by the Holy Spirit to become *makers* of peace.

For your sake and mine, I have to keep bringing us back to the bigger picture from the Lord's perspective. *Yes,* mending the broken spirit, surrendering, grieving, and reclaiming peace are necessary facets of healing what can never be erased from our personal stories. God's desire and design are indeed for our well-being. But we are not the point of our own stories! While forging a roadmap to wholeness is for our benefit, more importantly, it is an act of stewardship, and the inward work of transformation doesn't stop with us.

I get that you're exhausted. I know you want the storm clouds to pass. You're desperate for a break—for *peace.* But if the narrative you receive from me empowers you to stay limited inside the confines of the human condition, I haven't done my job. Behavior modification cannot change your heart. And if "your truth" doesn't lead you to *the* Truth, you'll just run in circles with every new wellness book that's released. Hear me clearly: Transformation is for wholeness, but wholeness is for strength, maturity, and longevity to serve the Lord and the people around us with humility, excellence, and honor—much like Joseph, Daniel, and Esther did in their respective generations.

By faith, lift your gaze above your circumstances and see the full salvation of the Lord at hand! Lay aside every burden that weighs you down. And as Isaiah prophesied, "Arise [from the depression and prostration in which circumstances have kept you—rise to a new life]! Shine (be radiant with the glory of the Lord), for your light has come, and the glory of the Lord has risen upon you!"[31] *Will you?* If your answer is yes, continue with me as we talk about how to cast our cares on the Lord. If your answer is no or "I'm not sure," stay with me still, because I believe the Lord is about to change your heart.

LAY YOUR BURDENS DOWN

In 1 Peter 5, we're given a roadmap to effectively offload our hearts' burdens on the Lord, which will ultimately lead to peace and maturity in character. The apostle Peter wrote,

> Clothe yourselves, all of you, with humility toward one another, for "God opposes the proud but gives grace to the humble."

Humble yourselves, therefore, under the mighty hand of God so that at the proper time he may exalt you, casting all your anxieties on him, because he cares for you. Be sober-minded; be watchful. Your adversary the devil prowls around like a roaring lion, seeking someone to devour. Resist him, firm in your faith, knowing that the same kinds of suffering are being experienced by your brotherhood throughout the world. And after you have suffered a little while, the God of all grace, who has called you to his eternal glory in Christ, will himself restore, confirm, strengthen, and establish you.[32]

Now, let's break this down. We know that perfect peace is the fruit of abiding in the Vine with a posture of trust and a fixed focus on the Lord. With that in mind, I'd like to propose that the framework of trust is built on the experience-based knowledge that we are loved unconditionally with perfect, complete love that drives out fear, fear that involves torment.[33] And this secure identity founded on perfect love conditions our hearts toward humility and dependence on the Lord's power, wisdom, and goodness in our lives.

Thus, through humility we embody the willing posture to cast our cares on Him, which leads to peace! Yet, it is a *lack* of trust that not only keeps us from transferring the weight of our burdens onto the Lord but also promotes the viability of an independent spirit that manifests pride and presumption—especially when we've chosen to separate ourselves from the Vine. And those two factors of the human personality are the ideal fare that a hungry Enemy is eager and primed to devour. When we release control (or rather, *the illusion* of control) to the Holy Spirit, we position ourselves in humility to receive the peace that passes all understanding. I truly believe this is why Paul wrote, "The peace of God, which surpasses all understanding, will guard your hearts and your minds in Christ Jesus."[34]

If unresolved pain from the past, aggravated afresh by an independent spirit, thwarts this perfect peace and trust, we will be fearful of what comes from the Lord. We will fear that His care and provision will be insufficient and disappointing. And in doing so, we will live at arm's length, in independence, leaning all the more on our own insight and understanding.

Do you now see why focus and trust through surrender, humility, and abiding in Him are critical for our livelihood? The orphan spirit is alive and well in too many believers today, and it is stealing our peace! Fear-based self-protection masquerades as strength and self-sufficiency in our false identities. Many of us have worn those false identities for so long that our true identities are indistinguishable, even to us. But today the Lord invites us into truth. And, yes, that truth is confrontational. However, the same truth that cuts also heals and leads us into freedom—spirit, soul, and body. We trust anyone to the extent we believe we are loved. Therefore, where we lack trust, we need to upgrade our awareness of His perfect love that drives out every trace of fear.

The apostle John wrote, "See what great love the Father has lavished on us, that we should be called children of God!"[35] Do *you* see it? Everything in life emanates from either fear or love. Out of perfect love, we trust and cast our cares. But out of fear, we hide in chaos and seek to control our lives. We need not abide there, however. Remember David who said, "The young lions suffer want and hunger; but *those who seek the LORD lack no good thing*."[36] With confidence, he also declared, "I believe that I shall look upon the goodness of the LORD in the land of the living! Wait for the LORD; be strong, and let your heart take courage; wait for the LORD!"[37] And it was Jesus who said,

I tell you, do not be anxious about your life, what you will eat or what you will drink, nor about your body, what you will put on. Is not life more than food, and the body more than clothing? Look at the birds of the air: they neither sow nor reap nor gather into barns, and yet your heavenly Father feeds them. Are you not of more value than they? And which of you by being anxious can add a single hour to his span of life? And why are you anxious about clothing? Consider the lilies of the field, how they grow: they neither toil nor spin, yet I tell you, even Solomon in all his glory was not arrayed like one of these. But if God so clothes the grass of the field, which today is alive and tomorrow is thrown into the oven, will he not much more clothe you, O you of little faith? Therefore do not be anxious, saying, "What shall we eat?" or "What shall we drink?" or "What shall we wear?" For the Gentiles seek after all these things, and your heavenly Father knows that you need them all. But seek first the kingdom of God and his righteousness, and all these things will be added to you.[38]

What great hope and assurance we have in Him! I pray that by these eternal, potent, God-breathed words, you will decide to lay down your penchant toward isolation, independence, self-preservation, and self-creation. And I pray that like the psalmist, you will enter the presence of the Lord fearlessly, confidently, and boldly,[39] saying to Him, "Unto You, O Lord, do I bring my life. O my God, I trust, lean on, rely on, and am confident in You. Let me not be put to shame or [my hope in You] be disappointed; let not my enemies triumph over me."[40]

Bring Him your *whole* life today. Lay every fear, doubt, disappointment, and insecurity at His feet. Rip off the mask. Throw off your outer garment, and receive today a robe of righteousness and a double portion instead of your shame.[41]

Are you sick and tired of striving to create peace and stability in your life? He will keep you in perfect peace as you keep your mind fixed and your heart trusting in Him, the One whose precious thoughts toward you outnumber the sand.[42] Receiving His peace isn't simply about resolving the surface-level responses to the pain in your life. It's about re-aiming the affections of your heart to King Jesus.

I want you to walk away from this chapter with a repeatable four-step process to offload the burdens of your heart as you fix your focus and re-anchor your trust in the Lord. Remember that casting your burdens isn't about closing loops. Nor is it about eliminating questions. It's about transferring the weight of your cares to the heart of the Lord, right in the midst of your uncertainty.

FOUR STEPS TO OFFLOAD YOUR BURDENS

Learning how to offload our burdens onto the Lord is a necessary rhythm we must develop for everyday life. Of course, Scripture provides a durable process to do exactly that:

1. **Come to Him.** In Matthew 11:28, Jesus said, "Come to me, all who labor and are heavy laden, and I will give you rest." The required action on our part is to come to Him— not in pretense but in truth, in transparency, and with our soul baggage, however weighty it is. This necessitates vulnerability and focus over time.

2. **Submit to Him.** There's no question that *submission* is a loaded word in our cultural context. Yet pure, godly submission is a call to yield our lives to the Lord, to defer to His direction and His ways. Moreover, submission requires the humility to admit that we're not great at running our own lives. As such, we must learn how to submit to His lordship. *Too many of us live as though He is Lord of some areas of life, but not Lord of all.* As we read earlier in the chapter, 1 Peter 5:5–6 says, "Clothe yourselves, all of you, with humility toward one another, for 'God opposes the proud but gives grace to the humble.' Humble yourselves, therefore, under the mighty hand of God so that at the proper time he may exalt you."

3. **Offload on Him.** Having humbled yourself before the Lord, you're now positioned to effectively offload your burdens onto His shoulders. First Peter 5:7 calls for "casting all your anxieties on him, because he cares for you." Notice that casting your anxieties comes *after* humbling

yourself. As a result of the posture of humility that says, "I need help because I have no idea what I'm doing here and am exhausted trying to control my life," you can release your cares without reservation and self-preservation. The psalmist galvanizes this sentiment in Psalm 55:22: "Cast your burden on the LORD, and he will sustain you; he will never permit the righteous to be moved."

4. **Receive from Him.** And when you offload your burdens to the Lord, the exchange occurs. Jesus said it this way in Matthew 11:29–30: "Take my yoke upon you, and learn from me, for I am gentle and lowly in heart, and you will find rest for your souls. For my yoke is easy, and my burden is light."

I understand the inherent challenge in this whole process. But that very fact is evidence of why we need to do away with our strong-willed proclivity to self-protect and go at life (and solve our problems) alone. An anxious heart will never know peace. Jesus's yoke is easy, and His burden is light. But you have to take it on yourself in humility and trust. In His presence is fullness of joy. In His presence, your soul is restored. So come to Him in truth today. Fix your focus. Anchor your heart in humble trust. And His perfect peace that passes all understanding will indeed be yours.

PERSONALIZE IT

THE POINT

Real peace is not a soul state absent of conflict; it is one that has been indwelled by the omnipotent presence of the Prince of Peace in every circumstance and trial.

THE PROMPT

In which area(s) of your life have you allowed adversity to occupy a greater place of focus than the Lord Himself? In which area(s) are you inclined to maintain independence and separateness? To hesitate to trust the steadfast character of the Lord? Why?

THE POSTURE

Perhaps the posture we need on the pathway to peace comes down to one word: *humility.* Humility calibrates our focus away from our circumstances and our dependence on ourselves toward our dependence on the Lord. Humility keeps us grounded in quiet, confident trust. And humility is the catalyst we need to come to Him, submit to Him, offload on Him, and receive from Him.

THE PRAYER

Lord, You said that Your yoke is easy and Your burden is light. I come to You to submit to You—to offload my burdens on You—that I might receive from You today. What would You have for me to receive, Lord? I'm tired of striving to create peace and stability in my life by my own strength. Whenever I'm inclined to assert my will to self-protect and take control of uncontrollable circumstances, help me to fix my focus on You. I receive Your peace right now, in Jesus's name. Amen.

NINE

CHECK THE GROUND

*Accordingly, the greatest need you and I have—
the greatest need of collective humanity—is
renovation of our heart.*

—DALLAS WILLARD, *Renovation of the Heart*

In chapter 2, I told you that while we can position ourselves for healing, I do not believe we can turn the key to systemic transformation in life by our own determination, desire, or will. That's perhaps most evident when we seemingly do the right things for change and growth but fail to experience the right results. Allow me to illustrate my point.

Some people have a great relationship with gardening. I don't. I tried to grow tomatoes once, then cucumbers. And when I fell in love with cooking, I attempted to grow other vegetables and even had a small herb garden. But if anyone is going to botch a garden, it's me. Despite that, I had an attractive plant at home for four years. I watered it once a week and made sure it had enough sunlight. I thought perhaps my streak of unintentional destruction was over. But in the last couple of months, I noticed that the leaves were starting to brown. So, I got out my scissors and went to town. To make matters worse, I didn't know you could overwater a plant. (Stop laughing. I told you this wasn't my gig.)

So, after chopping my plant down to size and nearly drowning it, I resolved to wait and watch for a week before considering the matter a lost cause. Well, a week came around quickly, and as you might expect, the plant had seen its last days. Overshadowed by a small cloud of remorse, I uprooted my formerly green friend and threw it in the trash. I really liked that plant too—not just because it was relatively easy to take care of but also because I enjoyed watching it grow and bloom, especially during the spring season here in Michigan.

But after taking a "gardening 101" deep dive on YouTube, I learned that what I failed to do was tend the soil. The seeds were obviously good. The sunlight was plentiful. And I stayed on top of providing enough water for the plant's growth. However, the ground needed to be tended to and loosened from time to time to break up the crusted soil. Suffice it to say, I learned my lesson. Despite the remarkable seeds I had at my disposal, long-term growth was contingent on the quality of the soil.

And right there is the reason I was stuck in an exhausting cycle of pain for two years. It's why you've been stuck too. You've done all the right things and applied the myriad of prescribed advice. Yet despite moderate change, the fruit of sustainable transformation is absent, isn't it? The problem in both of our cases is that we're looking in the wrong place for the change and growth we desire. So, having investigated the broken spirit, the insidious nature of shame, the art of surrender to the Lord for the work of transformation, the process of grief, and the pathway to peace, the next few chapters will be less about going wide and more about going deep. And that means we're headed straight for the heart.

> The output of our lives is wholly contingent on the interior health of our hearts.

You see, too many of us are frustrated, assuming that the problem exists with the seeds we're planting (meaning the valuable tools, resources, and relationships available to us) while simultaneously neglecting the soil into which those seeds are falling—namely, our hearts.

In Proverbs 4:23, Solomon wrote, "*Above all else,* guard your heart, for *everything* you do flows from it" (NIV). The New Living Translation offers a similar delivery: "Guard your heart above all else, for it *determines the course of your life.*" And just to thread the needle through this point, *The Message* paraphrase of the same verse reads, "Keep vigilant watch over your heart; *that's* where life starts."[1]

In other words, just like the quality of the soil determines the fruitfulness of the seed, the output of our lives is wholly contingent on the interior health of our hearts. But our overfamiliarity with that verse has prevented many of us from pausing to ask the question that is key to unlocking and catalyzing inside-out life transformation. It's a simple question too: *What, according to Scripture, is the heart?*

THE HEART-MIND CONNECTION

Most of us probably designate the heart as the seat of our emotions and the brain as the physical location of the mind, right? But when the Bible was written, there was no such separation.

In Proverbs 4:23, originally written in Hebrew, the word translated "heart" emanates from the word *lêb,* which the *Brown-Driver-Briggs Hebrew and English Lexicon* defines as the "inner man, mind, will, heart" and relates to such concepts as the soul; knowledge; "inclinations, resolutions and determinations of the will"; and the "seat of the emotions."[2] *Strong's Exhaustive Concordance* describes *lêb* as "used (figuratively) very widely for the feelings, the will and even the intellect."[3] The New Testament equivalent is the Koine Greek word *kardia,* which is the etymological origin of modern English words for things pertaining to our physical hearts. It refers to "the soul or *mind,* as it is the fountain and *seat of the thoughts,* passions, desires, appetites, affections, purposes, endeavors; . . . the understanding, the faculty and seat of intelligence; . . . the will and character . . . of the soul so far forth as it is affected and stirred in a bad way or good."[4]

In effect, we have just described the *soul,* which is the aggregate of one's rational mind and intellect, seat of emotions, and determination and will. Returning to the metaphor of seeds and soil, the soil is the heart, and the heart includes the mind. It's no wonder Solomon wrote, "As he thinks in his heart, so is he."[5] This means that we see the world not as it is but *as we are* in our thoughts, in our affections, and in the totality of our inner beings.

For some of us, the health of our hearts might produce confidence and hope even amid pain and heartbreak. But if you're like me and have unintentionally nurtured a measure of ungrieved loss, bitterness, or unresolved disappointment—or have not brought healing to a significant traumatic memory in your life—not one positive seed will harvest until you first deal with the diseased, distressed soil of your heart.

When I gained this insight through my own studies and in counseling, it was a breakthrough moment. In fact, when it happened, I began to sense another layer of hope rise in my heart. This single thread on the tapestry of trauma, pain, shame, and blame I'd worn for years began to unravel. And in its slow unraveling, I became relentless in my pursuit of wholeness.

Guarding the affections of our hearts is a preeminent need as we forge our roadmaps to wholeness. Validating the need for this crucial work, Dallas Willard, in his classic *Renovation of the Heart,* wrote, "A carefully cultivated heart will, assisted by the grace of God, foresee, forestall, or transform most of the painful situations before which others stand like helpless children saying 'Why?'" He continued, "Accordingly, the greatest need you and I have— the greatest need of collective humanity—is *renovation of our heart. . . .* Indeed, the only hope of humanity lies in the fact that, as our spiritual dimension has been *formed,* so it also can be *transformed.*"[6] His words have reverberated through my spirit for years and are thus the reason we must proceed further into our investigation of the heart.

The Divided Heart

As a consequence of our living out of wounded souls and broken spirits, the unresolved issues of our hearts will distract us from truth, divide our focus from the present moment, and distort our perception of reality. Inevitably, pain, shame, loss, bitterness, pride, and even self-centeredness not only become lenses through which we see life but also act

> Pain makes a terrible compass.

as compasses for our daily activities. And one thing is sure: Pain makes a terrible compass.

Jesus illustrated this point in Matthew 13:22, when he said, "As for what was sown among thorns, this is the one who hears the word, but the *cares of the world* and the deceitfulness of riches *choke* the word, and it proves *unfruitful.*" While the obvious context of this verse is a person who is lured by the pleasure and delight of riches, the underlying principle speaks of the trappings of a distracted, divided heart. This is evidence for why we'll never find sustained victory in life without first dealing with the underlying issues of the heart.

I want to unpack this verse a bit more to fortify my point. The Greek word for "care" here is *merimna,* which can also mean "anxiety."[7] But most interestingly, the root word of *merimna* is the verb *merizo,* which means "to divide into parties, i.e., be split into factions."[8]

Thus, a divided heart (illustrated by the thorny soil in Jesus's parable) is not calibrated to the present. Instead, when our hearts' affections are attuned to either the pain of the past or the uncertainty of the future, where trauma and anxiety rule and reign, our divided hearts will prevent us from living with a single focused purpose for life.

It was Jesus who said, "The eye is the lamp of the body. So, if your eye is healthy, your whole body will be full of light."[9] Again, in context, He was teaching His disciples about not stockpiling treasures here on Earth. But in a broader sense, He was saying that when the metaphorical eyes of our hearts are free of distraction and unencumbered by the weight of our cares, our life focus, our hearts' affections, and our decisions will be established aright from a place of wholeness. It's precisely why Jesus demonstrated that the quality of the soil *always* determines the fruitfulness of the seed. And in doing so, He elevated the game to another level of intensity.

CHECK THE GROUND

The gospel of Mark chapter 4 is one of my favorite portions of Scripture—not only because the principles therein are central to the theme of this book but also because it provided a framework for my journey to transformation and wholeness. In fact, it's so central to Jesus's teaching that in verse 13, He said, "Do you not understand this parable? How then will you understand all the parables?" In other words, if you don't understand this one, you won't understand any of the others. It's that big of a deal. Let's pick up with Jesus in verses 3–9:

> "Listen! Behold, a sower went out to sow. And as he sowed, some seed fell along the path, and the birds came and devoured it. Other seed fell on rocky ground, where it did not have much soil, and immediately it sprang up, since it had no depth of soil. And when the sun rose, it was scorched, and since it had no root, it withered away. Other seed fell among thorns, and the thorns grew up and choked it, and it yielded no grain. And other seeds fell into good soil and produced grain, growing up and increasing and yielding thirtyfold and sixtyfold and a hundredfold." And he said, "He who has ears to hear, let him hear."

In this passage, Jesus identified soil of four different qualities. The same kind of seed was planted in each one, but the results were drastically different. Why? Because as you now understand, you can have the best seeds available, but if you plant them in bad soil, you're not going to reap good fruit. This is precisely why willpower-driven self-help, let alone the self-healing narrative, cannot produce what only transformation by the Holy Spirit will do.

In my own life, I was planting all the right seeds for growth, but I failed to initially deal with the core issues of my heart in the process: the perpetual negative emotions, unresolved disappointment, bitterness, and traumatic memories, most certainly including regret from my past. As a result, the overriding disposition of my soul and spirit was drowning in brokenness, pain, fear, and shame. So, no matter how many good seeds I "threw into the soil," my creativity was stifled, my long-term growth suffered, and the people closest to me knew it.

Yet beyond convenience and comfort, Jesus made an even stronger case for wholeness and healing the issues of the heart: Not only does living from wounded spirits and souls hamper our best efforts, but the infertility of diseased, distracted hearts also strangles the effective power of the Word of God. Please understand that this is not because of the vulnerability or fragility of the Word itself. Rather, it is because the quality of the soil determines the success of the seed planted within.

This is a key principle for the entire book—one that validates the limitations of our own determination, as we discussed in chapter 2: The Word of God *itself* contains the power to confront, cut, clean, and heal that which hinders us from living a life of wholeness. Not willpower. Not self-help. Not self-healing. Yet the strength of the Word is limited by our level of surrender to, and cooperation with, the work of the Holy Spirit in our lives.

Regarding the Word's inherent strength, Hebrews 4:12 says, "The word of God is living and active, sharper than any two-edged sword, piercing to the division of soul and of spirit, of joints and of marrow, and discerning the thoughts and intentions of the heart." James 1:21–22 validates this, admonishing us to "put away all filthiness and rampant wickedness and receive with meekness the implanted word, which is able to save your souls. But be doers of the word, and not hearers only, deceiving yourselves." Still, the last part of that verse reveals the underlying reason why many of us hear the Word; set our intentions to make changes so we can move through pain and loss, disappointment and grief; yet still come up short in our pursuit of healing and wholeness.

> The Word of God *itself* contains the power to confront, cut, clean, and heal that which hinders us from living a life of wholeness. Not willpower. Not self-help. Not self-healing.

Truthfully, it's embarrassing to admit that more than once in the past several years, I've unintentionally (and maybe even intentionally) sabotaged my own growth. We all are baited to do the same. But why do we do it? Why do we, as James warned, betray ourselves "into deception by reasoning contrary to the Truth"?[10] Because the drive for control and independence after pain and loss, combined with the subsequent fear of losing *more* control of our perceived fragile and disconnected lives, has insulated and isolated us inside the prison of our hardened hearts.

WHY WE DON'T CHANGE

It's precisely what happened to the children of Israel. Remember from chapter 3 that although they had been delivered from the bondage of slavery, "slavery" never got out of them. They were living out of broken spirits. For forty years, they witnessed abundant provision from the Lord, yet throughout their journey, they complained and became bitter toward Him. What they experienced in Egypt *happened*, but it wasn't currently *happening*. Yet their embittered hearts, hardened by self-protection and self-promotion and anchored in the toxicity of unbelief, cut them off from receiving life and provision through dependence on the Father. Just like it did for me.

What happened to me *happened*. But it wasn't presently *happening*. And until I was willing to own the parts of my story that

I never wanted to revisit—until I regularly uprooted and confronted the diseased, fear-based issues of the soil of my heart—what remained were unhealed skeletons. They were grim memorials of loss that validated my drive for independence and control. "Because if He really loved me, if He *really cared* about me," I vehemently contended, "my mom would still be alive today and my body wouldn't have broken down and betrayed me at a time when I needed strength the most."

And that just might be your story too.

While I cannot stand face-to-face with you in this moment, I want to plead with you to not let another day go by without taking the first step toward opening the doors of your own dark, isolated prison of the past. What happened, *happened*. And I'm so sorry for that. But it may not be happening still.

I am not telling you to rush through the process of grieving your losses. Though you never have to move *on* from what happened, you must move *forward* if you want to be whole. Had the children of Israel chosen to move forward, their memorial of loss might have more quickly become a testimony of redemption. Let's take a closer look at their state of affairs.

The writer of Hebrews gives us an eyewitness account of their exact situation. Hebrews 3:8–11 says:

> Do not harden your hearts as in the rebellion,
>   on the day of testing in the wilderness,
> where your fathers put me to the test
>   and saw my works for forty years.
> Therefore I was provoked with that generation,
> and said, "They always go astray in their heart;
>   they have not known my ways."
> As I swore in my wrath,
>   "They shall not enter my rest."

Right there in verse 10 is why the children of Israel persisted in their hardened state: They went astray in their hearts. Though their past was true, it wasn't the truth about their promised future.

Too many of us, myself included, have labeled our true, valid, painful life experiences as *truth* concerning the trajectory of the rest of our lives, and that has to stop! It's a shortsighted rip-off of our purpose. If I could put a target for this principle in the cross-hairs, it would be this: The devastating by-product of living from wounded souls and broken spirits is that our chosen path of independence separates us from our awareness of and experience with the goodness of the Lord. And it is this goodness of the Lord, inherent to His nature, that offers rest, hope, and redemption for our weary souls.

In the next chapter, we'll leverage two helpful tools as we learn how to work the ground of our hearts. Then in chapter 11, we will investigate the power of a transformed mind.

PERSONALIZE IT

THE POINT

The quality of the soil determines the fruitfulness of the seed. In other words, the output of our lives is wholly contingent on the interior health of our hearts.

THE PROMPT

What is the current state of your heart? Is it hardened and offended? Hurt? Jaded? Cynical? Unbelieving? Distracted? Afraid? Or is it healthy and whole? What event or circumstance provoked this heart condition? Take an audit of the condition of your heart right now. What adjustments do you need to make in life so you no longer perpetuate and normalize those conditions but address them, deal with them, and move forward?

THE POSTURE

What proactive measures will you take to ensure that you don't go astray in your heart like the children of Israel? These can be very practical decisions. Consider Solomon's wisdom once again: "Guard your heart above all else, for it determines the course of your life."[11]

THE PRAYER

Lord, Your Word is clear about the necessary priority to keep and guard my heart above everything else in my life. So today, I ask You to help me maintain that priority. I invite Your Word to confront, cut, clean, and heal that which is hindering me from living a life of wholeness. My desire is to live undistracted and undivided in my heart toward You. I want to enter Your rest. Amen.

TEN

WORK THE GROUND

A calm and undisturbed mind and heart are the life and health of the body, but envy, jealousy, and wrath are like rottenness of the bones.

—PROVERBS 14:30, AMPC

Let me take you back to the cycle of pain I shared in chapter 3 to reinforce the severity of the consequences of living in this dilapidated soul state long-term. As we discussed earlier, the neurobiological reflex connected to chronic stress, unresolved pain, unhealed wounds, and ungrieved loss following trauma is self-protection, which in effect tries to insulate the heart from future pain.

And while that makes sense from a survival perspective, it isn't healthy in a chronic state. "Allostasis," according to Elizabeth Stanley, "allows us to mobilize the appropriate amount of energy and focus for coping well before, during, and after the threat or challenge. However, with *chronic* or *prolonged stress,* our mind-body system doesn't complete a full recovery after a stressful experience—instead, it remains in an activated state." Moreover, "trauma can occur if, during a stressful experience, we also perceive ourselves to be *powerless, helpless,* or *lacking control.* Trauma is especially likely to result if aspects of the current threat or challenge contain cues or triggers related to traumatic events from earlier in our lives."[1] That's *exactly* why I stayed stuck in a cycle of pain, shame, and blame longer than I needed to. And it's precisely the destructive path the children of Israel took, as we read in Hebrews 3:10: "They always go astray in their heart; they have not known my ways."

How, then, do our hearts lead us astray just like theirs? Our dysfunctional dispositions cause us to make faulty judgments about the safety, reliability, and intentions of the people closest to us—most especially about the Lord Himself. We make these judgments because circumstances appear to validate our perception that we are indeed, as Stanley articulated, "powerless, helpless, or lacking control."[2] In so doing, we inevitably construct a victim mentality through which we live our everyday lives.

Following this train down the tracks, over time, the repeated behavior of self-protection leads to isolation, fostering separateness in our hearts, which ultimately suffocates and atrophies our connection to Life Himself. This then breaks our spirits and renders us stuck, defeated, hopeless, and physically sick. Bessel van der Kolk brings physiological credence to this biblical truth:

> Constantly fighting unseen dangers is exhausting and leaves [people who have experienced trauma] fatigued, depressed, and weary. If elements of the trauma are replayed again and again, the accompanying stress hormones engrave those memories ever more deeply in the mind. Ordinary, day-to-day events become less and less compelling. Not being able to deeply take in what is going on around them makes it *impossible to feel fully alive*. . . . Not being fully alive in the present keeps them *more firmly imprisoned in the past*.[3]

I've said it before: Though the children of Israel got out of Egypt, "Egypt" never got out of them. In fact, I want you to take a moment to canvass your life right now. Ask yourself, *What's my "Egypt"?* Maybe you've been distant from that loss, sickness, defeat, relationship betrayal, untimely death, or financial collapse for years now, but the weight of the experience still lies across your heart today. Worse, maybe the roots in the soil of your heart stem all the way back to childhood. Again, I am not making light or being dismissive of your circumstance, but wouldn't you agree that the imprisonment of the past is certainly no place to dwell any longer? The choice to position ourselves for healing and transformation is one we must make each day.

As I'm writing this chapter, I'm in a decent amount of physical pain. Dealing with an autoimmune disease like multiple sclerosis is interesting because from the outside, people see my smile, but beneath the smile today is an aching body. Don't get me wrong, though. Overall, I'm doing fantastic, but today is the fifth day in a row of low, dark clouds here in metro Detroit, a peculiarity for mid-July. Mix in the cocktail of heat and humidity, and all I want to do is lie on the couch, because this weather is a key trigger for MS flares. On the phone yesterday, I told a friend that writing this book has been the one of the hardest things I've ever done—not because I'm struggling to convey my thoughts but because my present physical pain cracks the seal on depression and anxiety, which taunt me to not believe the very words I'm writing. Oh, in these moments, I can hear the cynics, skeptics, disappointed, and disillusioned shout in accusation, "Where is the faithfulness of your God and the reliability of His character today?" It's there. *I know it's there.* I've seen an immeasurable portion of His faithfulness in my life too often to turn back now.

Psalm 20:1 says, "May the LORD answer you in the day of trouble! May the name of the God of Jacob protect you!" *Today* is the day of salvation. And if I don't feel better today, when tomorrow becomes "today," I'll still attend to the truth of His Word. This is the power of a fixed focus. I don't simply believe *in* the Lord. I believe *Him.* I believe every word He has spoken. My job is to deliver this message to you with authenticity. And authenticity isn't doing what feels right; authenticity is doing what is right. It's precisely why moving forward through pain and moving on from pain are vastly different experiences.

You never have to take an eraser to a treacherous season of your life. Ever. "Moving on" demands amnesia about your past—and that's utter nonsense. But if you want to experience wholeness and redemption, moving forward through pain and etched with scars is a nonnegotiable choice. For that reason, we must commit to showing up in the truth of what happened and where we are in life today. The early traumatic memories of our past *must* experience healing by the power of the Holy Spirit, because without it, we're involuntarily charting a course whose navigational devices are fear, pain, shame, blame, and victimhood.

This is why the quality of the soil always determines the fruitfulness of the seed. *This* is why the output of our lives is wholly dependent on the interior health of our hearts. *This* is why we must determine to not find sufficiency for life in our deficiencies. Because of unexposed and unhealed wounds, we unintentionally normalize mindsets and behaviors that are anything but normal. In fact, the very things we see as not only helpful but also *necessary* to keep ourselves safe, powerful, and *in control* are the same mindsets and behaviors that actually destroy our essence from the inside out.

I'm so sick and tired of being sick and tired. How about you? It's time to be *doers* and *producers* of the Word. It's time, my friend, to work the ground of our hearts.

WORK THE GROUND

I want to equip you with various practical strategies to deal with the deep-seated issues of your heart on a regular basis, so that you aren't unintentionally frustrating yourself by your own habitual, learned devices. But my greatest aim is to help you learn to become more aware of your heart issues in the first place—issues that will prevent you from assimilating the strength of the Word into your spirit, soul, and body by the power of the Holy Spirit.

Maturity should be the target of every believer, and we are responsible for the stewardship of our lives. Therefore, we must take responsibility for our own health and growth. This was Paul's charge in 1 Thessalonians 5:23: "May the God of peace himself sanctify you completely, and may your whole spirit and soul and body be kept blameless at the coming of our Lord Jesus Christ." It doesn't mean we are responsible for the growth itself; rather, when it comes to the outworking of our lives of wholeness, it is up to us to position ourselves for effective partnership with the Lord.[4] That is, if we're ever going to experience change in life, we have to first own our stuff.

In October 2014, when I was at a pivotal breaking point, I most certainly did not receive immediate or overnight breakthrough. But what I did receive was a seed: an opportunity to begin the process of a "walk through" into healing. When the Lord asked me, "What do you want Me to do for you?" I knew He was asking because my partnership would be required for healing. I had to take responsibility for *where I was* and *what happened* before I could take one step forward into *what was possible.*

He is both a God of breakthrough and a God of process. And because faith requires action, I did what seemed like the only thing I could do: cry out for help. I was ready to get to work but didn't know how or where to start. Moreover, I was exhausted and, to be honest, a little annoyed that I couldn't simply go to sleep and wake up completely healed. And while breakthrough is incredible—and *real*—"walk through" was the designated route for me. It would build necessary muscles of perseverance and enduring faith within my soul. Would there be scars along the way? You bet. But hear me clearly: The presence of scars in any area of life tells a story whose end is healing and restoration.

Your scars, like mine, tell a story—perhaps of pain and loss but also about the reliability of our God. Comfort is not simply what He does; *Comforter* is who He is.

In the heat of my battle, I memorized Psalm 68:19, and each morning and evening, I looked in the mirror at the exhausted, tear-stained face staring back at me and commanded my soul, "Blessed be the Lord, Who bears [*my*] burdens and carries [*me*] day by day, even the God Who is [*my*] salvation!" (AMPC). That verse not only carried me through most days in late 2012 and throughout 2013 but also served as a constant reminder that my responsibility was *today.* And while I was growing *today,* He was doing the heavy lifting of my burdens and carrying me faithfully in His grace and presence, so long as I was willing to show up.

I hope that encourages you in your own journey. I want to galvanize the idea of what it means to be responsible for today by taking it from theory into practice, because we cannot fix or heal ourselves *in and of* ourselves.

A couple of years ago, I developed an interdependent rhythm that has paid tremendous dividends to my mental, emotional, and spiritual well-being. It's called "posture, then practice."

Posture

I don't know what I don't know. I just don't have it in me to thoroughly change my life in my own strength or even desire. That's why I'm thoroughly convinced that willpower-driven self-help *helps* but will not catalyze sustainable transformation of spirit, soul, and body in any of our lives. And as I said earlier, just because something may be true in life doesn't mean it is the truth. So, before we head into any direction of heart work or inner healing, we must make sure the compasses of our hearts and spirits are set on truth: the Spirit of Truth Himself who will lead and guide us into all truth.[5] Indeed, He is the One who called us by name before the foundation of the earth. Remember the psalmist's words:

> O LORD, you have searched me and known me!
> You know when I sit down and when I rise up;
>   you discern my thoughts from afar.
> You search out my path and my lying down
>   and are acquainted with all my ways.
> Even before a word is on my tongue,
>   behold, O LORD, you know it altogether.
> You hem me in, behind and before,
>   and lay your hand upon me.
> Such knowledge is too wonderful for me;
>   it is high; I cannot attain it.
>
> Where shall I go from your Spirit?
>   Or where shall I flee from your presence?

If I ascend to heaven, you are there!
    If I make my bed in Sheol, you are there!
If I take the wings of the morning
    and dwell in the uttermost parts of the sea,
even there your hand shall lead me,
    and your right hand shall hold me. . . .

For you formed my inward parts;
    you knitted me together in my mother's womb.
I praise you, for I am fearfully and wonderfully made.
Wonderful are your works;
    my soul knows it very well.
My frame was not hidden from you,
when I was being made in secret,
    intricately woven in the depths of the earth.
Your eyes saw my unformed substance;
in your book were written, every one of them,
    the days that were formed for me,
    when as yet there was none of them.

How precious to me are your thoughts, O God!
    How vast is the sum of them![6]

And in great consequence of this beautiful reality, the *posture* from which I *practice* the deep work of healing the soil of my heart is this, a prayer from the same pen that wrote the psalm above:

Search me, O God, and know my heart!
    Try me and know my thoughts!
And see if there be any grievous way in me,
    and lead me in the way everlasting![7]

By calibrating my heart "due north" toward the Lord, I invited Him to crash my independence and strong will with His presence that both cuts and exposes but also heals and restores what is broken. In the same motion, my proverbially bloodied fists of battle could finally drop from their on-guard position in the safety of God's presence, where neither self-protection nor self-promotion was needed for survival.

And know this: *Posture always precedes practice.* It's a necessary principle to understand, for posture establishes the aim and focus of our minds and hearts away from independence and control and toward dependence on the Spirit of the Lord and the rock-solid foundation of His Word. In turn, the Holy Spirit will fill us with the truth and tools to uproot the malignancies of our souls and thus cast aside every weight that so easily ensnares us.[8] Practice without posture probably explains the futility of willpower, too, because central to its ideological framework is the notion that the strength and strategies to change start *and end* with us. And one thing's for sure: We can't fix or heal ourselves. I tried for too long, and while the effort was understandable and perhaps even a good try, it was bound to frustrate me and fail from the outset. Posture, then practice is the movement from independence to dependence on the Holy Spirit for what we need most: transformation from the inside out, which far outperforms behavior modification.

Practically speaking, establishing my posture is a regular practice in which I simply pray words similar to those in Psalm 139: "Search me and know me. . . . Try . . . weigh . . . investigate my thoughts and attitudes, Lord." Then I'll take a moment to wait on Him and listen, and I encourage you to do the same. Be sure to have a notebook or a notes app available so you can keep record of what the Lord reveals to you. This simple exercise aids the development of a "hearing ear," which I believe is a cornerstone to our spiritual formation. And as the Lord speaks, quickly obey. Follow His lead with a spirit of humility. This regular act of faithful dependence on the Lord (the posture of those whom Jesus called "poor in spirit" in Matthew 5:3)[9] positions us to audit the condition of our hearts, make adjustments, and thus walk in the maturity and wholeness to which we are called.

PRACTICE

Having established the posture from which we'll work the ground of our hearts, I would like to share two primary tools I use to carry out that intention. The first is regular self-awareness with applied self-knowledge. And the second is a guided exercise using emotions as "flashlights" to expose deeper, more insidious areas of a wounded soul. Both activities are best experienced in the presence and counsel of a wise teacher, mentor, pastor, or professional counselor, because navigating difficult past hurts and even painful emotions is sometimes hard to do—let alone effective or even wise—when we're going at it alone.

Let's explore the first tool in our groundwork toolbox: self-awareness.

Tool #1: Self-Awareness

Self-awareness with applied self-knowledge is an incredibly helpful exercise to use as you begin this deep work. Fundamentally, self-awareness is an honest understanding of yourself: your personal habits and strengths, as well as areas where you need improvement, and your way of perceiving life. In simple fashion, self-awareness is about acknowledging "Yes, this happened (or is happening)" or "Yes, I did (or am doing) this."

But what turns the key on self-awareness is applied self-knowledge. If self-awareness is the *what* of our situation, then self-knowledge is the *why*—our underlying motivation. When we can look in the mirror and admit, "Yes, I'm in a lot of pain. Yes, I'm stuck. And, yes, life is moving forward but I'm not" and then begin exploring *why* we're not progressing, we will effectively turn a necessary key to personal transformation.

You see, while acknowledging the pain and loss I had experienced was important, leveraging that self-awareness with applied self-knowledge then allowed me to admit that I was living stuck and examine why I was justifying that mindset and behavior. And *that part* was my choice. The Lord knew I was stuck. My friends and family knew I was stuck. But until I was willing to confront my own reality with both truth and compassion, I could not correct the course of my life.

This is the power of confession—truth telling, as we talked about in chapter 6. Until our *true* collides with *the* Way, *the* Truth, and *the* Life Himself, we will live in a perpetual cycle of being stuck. How true that was for me and how true that is for you too. Interestingly, the potency of self-awareness isn't restricted to our minds alone. Elizabeth Stanley illuminated the neurobiological power of awareness:

> *Awareness* does not belong to the thinking brain or the survival brain. It functions distinct from the thinking brain's cognitive activity and the survival brain's stress and emotional arousal. Awareness is greater than all of these things— which is why we can pay attention to thoughts, emotions, physical sensations, and the body's posture, temperature, and movements. Mindfulness-based training helps us learn how to *direct and sustain our attention—and thereby stabilize awareness*—so that we can become aware of, learn from, and modulate these different mind-body experiences.[10]

In stabilizing awareness, I believe we are doing the necessary work of unburdening the soil of our hearts for future healing and wholeness. But there is a catch to this utility of self-awareness: We can't see what we can't see. We all have blind spots in various areas of life. Therefore, one of the most effective and honest ways to develop both self-awareness and self-knowledge is to invite feedback into your life from a trusted mentor. Ask them, "What do you know about me that I don't know and need to know?" Then get ready to listen. Now, hear me out: This exercise isn't one of self-deprecation. Instead, it's an honest growth tactic to keep you from living stuck in self-sabotaging, self-destructive patterns of dysfunction.

A key benefit of inviting feedback into your life is that it keeps your "knife" sharp, so to speak. Allow me to explain. As a pretty serious home cook, I take great care of my kitchen equipment, especially my knives. And the most dangerous knife in my arsenal is the dullest knife—the one that has not met an adequate amount of abrasion, or conflict, with a sharpening stone. That's exactly the function of often abrasive, unpleasant, confrontational feedback in our own lives. Indeed, "faithful are the wounds of a friend"![11] Few of us enjoy hard conversations, and perhaps fewer eagerly pursue the pain of change that leads to transformation. But I'd like to propose that developing the maturity of character to step into difficult conversations keeps us sharp and effective as we meet the challenges of everyday life and move through our pain into purpose.

Tool #2: Emotions as Flashlights

Another helpful tool I've learned and employed over the last several years is to utilize emotions—*however* and *whenever* they show up—as flashlights to illuminate more consequential and systemic areas of fear, shame, guilt, bitterness, or regret in my heart, as well as any unhealed soul wounds, unresolved disappointments, and ungrieved losses. Emotions themselves are not good or bad,[12] though we often recognize them as being pleasant or unpleasant. Instead, they're quite valuable for personal growth, especially when we name them, which reduces the intensity of their presence in the moment.

And accompanying those emotions are thoughts, often sewn together by beliefs and determinations we've made about ourselves in light of our past experiences. Sadly, though, those deep-seated beliefs typically manifest in subconscious self-sabotaging identity statements such as "Because [this event] happened, I am therefore [false identity label]." Let's use the emotion of anger to paint a picture of a familiar scene.

THE ISSUE BEHIND THE ISSUE

It's Tuesday morning, and even after a nice (but quick) weekend and a less-than-hectic Monday, you've noticed an unusual bent toward anger over the past week—so much so, that a slow, steady drip of caffeinated irritation is pervading your day. Why? Who knows, but there's no time to figure that out now. It's eight o'clock and you've already spilled the coffee and yelled at the dog for making you spill the coffee that was never good to begin with. The weather's supposed to be hot and humid today, and you just remembered that you forgot to turn on the AC before you left the house. *Great.* Oh, and you forgot to put gas in the car last night. *Traffic had better be light.*

At this point, the podcast on the drive into the office just adds to the noise, though somehow, hitting pause doesn't stop the chatter inside your head. *Here it comes.* You can feel it in your clenched jaw and tightened shoulders. It's the braced posture as you walk to your desk. And just as the pinch before the throb of another headache arrives, you realize your coffee's now cold and the ibuprofen bottle is empty. The kindling that stokes the flame in your soul, of course, is an ornery email from a coworker and the app notification of the missed delivery of an expected important package.

By late afternoon, you're ready to wave the white flag. As if on cue, your phone buzzes with hurried and perceived sharp words from your significant other. Something about a puddle of coffee on the countertop and chicken that was supposed to be for dinner but is still in the freezer. *But don't worry; it's only Tuesday.* Eyeing the weekend with surrendered intensity, you're reminded of the feverish pace of a busy life that's producing nothing more than an end-of-the-week crash and a laundry list of . . . laundry . . . and wishes for a different life.

You've been there, right? We all have those days when irritation turned anger seems to run the show and won't let go. But when once-in-a-while days turn into regular weeks, weeks into months, and months into a "new normal" that's anything but normal, we need to make a quick, concerted effort to confront the underlying thoughts and mindsets, enflamed by emotions, that are navigating the direction of our souls . . . which in this case is anger.

Anger in and of itself is a normal emotion in our human condition. We're all flawed, and life is messy. But it's never *really* about the coffee, the dog, the AC, the chicken, or the email, is it? It's always about the issue behind the issue. That's what this practice is about: exposing and excavating the issues of the heart that affect all we do and all we are. When we leverage the presence of anger to explore and expose the deeper motivating issue, we often uncover the insidious presence of resentment, humiliation, disappointment, and even a feeling of disrespect that cascades across a variety of circumstances and relationships.

THOUGHTS AND EMOTIONS
ALWAYS WORK TOGETHER

Of great importance, "notice that feeling and thought always go together," Dallas Willard wrote. "They are interdependent and are never found apart. There is no feeling without something being before the mind in thought and no thought without some positive or negative feeling toward what is contemplated."[13] Therefore, the emotion leads us to the thought, where the neurobiological ability to steer our behaviors and thus determine our actions resides.

But we're not finished yet. Digging deeper, underneath those thoughts are mindsets and beliefs that reside in (and play back) from the subconscious, and they drive the majority of our everyday lives. In my journey to wholeness, when I used the presence of anger in my life as a flashlight, it revealed resentment and humiliation that expressed themselves as irritation or frustration and caused me to withdraw from tense situations and, sadly, sometimes harbor a critical spirit against others. But beneath the resentment and humiliation, I discovered a faulty, diseased belief that emanated from childhood—the primary core issue and malady in the soil of my heart that stifled my growth and health for too long: *It's not that I made a mistake or even that others have made mistakes. I am a mistake. If I wasn't me, this situation wouldn't have happened. There is something intrinsically wrong with me. I, in and of myself, am defective. The outcome of my performance dictates my worth. It always has and always will.*

This kind of default narrative, core belief, or false identity, based in fear, informs the thoughts that motivate our behavior, steering the course of our lives down unfavorable paths. (We'll explore this much more in the next chapter.) It's the diseased root that ruins the soil of our hearts, choking the life out of any seed that falls on it. And it is precisely why the quality of the soil always determines the fruitfulness of the seed.

Most importantly, though, this exercise of using our emotions as flashlights is not simply for wellness; it's our righteous requirement as sons and daughters of the King. Exposing and excavating the issues of our hearts isn't so much about self-care as about conforming to His will and His purpose for us—and enabling the total transformation of our spirits, souls, and bodies by the renewal of our minds.[14]

This weightier eternal perspective was established when the apostle Paul wrote in Ephesians 4:21–27:

> You . . . were taught . . . to put off your old self, which belongs to your former manner of life and is corrupt through deceitful desires, and to be renewed in the spirit of your minds, and to put on the new self, created after the likeness of God in true righteousness and holiness. Therefore, having put away falsehood, let each one of you speak the truth with his neighbor, for we are members one of another. Be angry and do not sin; do not let the sun go down on your anger, and give no opportunity to the devil.

That's what this practice of working the ground is all about: exposing and excavating issues of the heart left unchecked. And we do this by paying attention to the pervading presence of negative emotions whose roots are toxic thoughts and destructive mindsets. It's these very issues that push us toward fear and isolation—and, as a result, a life of independence (separateness) and the drive to control. But when we show up and do the work, in complete dependence on the Holy Spirit's power, we recognize and reject false identities and sin patterns that ensnare us in a life void of abiding love, trust, surrender, and transformation that lead to wholeness.

A TOOL FOR PRACTICE

As you engage in the posture and practice of working the ground of your heart with your mentor, counselor, or pastor, a useful accessory is the Feeling Wheel.[15] It is a simple display of emotions common to all of us, with a subset of inciting emotions that allow us to put language to the deeper issues of the heart. To access this free, helpful tool, follow the link I've provided in the endnotes.

A GUIDED EXERCISE

Now I'm going to lead you through a guided exercise of using pervasive negative emotions as flashlights to help you identify underlying destructive false beliefs that are steering your life.[16] Please write your findings down and take them into a coaching or counseling session so that your mentor can help reflect your discoveries back to you, in the presence of the Lord, while weighing them against Scripture. This is crucial because perspective and transformation take place when we compare our true lived experiences with the anchor of the truth, which is the Word of God. We may feel led in a particular direction, but unless it lines up with the principles expressed and confirmed through the Scriptures, we need to hold our findings relatively loosely. I say that from a heart of great passion for people to grow in maturity unto the Lord.

So, ready yourself with a notebook and a pen or the notes app on your phone. Find a comfortable place to sit where you can work through the exercise unhurried. But first, let's pray together. Join me out loud:

Father, I come before You in the name of Jesus. I believe, according to Your Word, that Jesus took stripes not only for my healing but also for my wholeness, spirit, soul, and body.

And so today, Lord, I ask You to search me and know me. Try, weigh, and investigate my thoughts and attitudes, Lord. I give You access to every self-protected, isolated, fearful place of my heart. I know, even in this moment, though it might be scary, that You're with me. I believe You've redeemed my life from destruction, so, Lord, my life is Yours. I want to experience health and wholeness in my mind, body, and spirit so I can live in my true identity, free of fear and in Your perfect love. I ask that You silence the taunts of the Enemy in this moment so that Your Holy Spirit is the only voice I hear. Speak to me today. In Jesus's name, amen.

And now . . .

1. **What is a dominant negative emotion you experience on a regular basis?**

   If you need assistance, utilize the Feeling Wheel I referenced earlier. Write your answer down. Is there a secondary emotion behind this emotion? (Use the Feeling Wheel as a prompt.)

2. **Now, take some time to think about a recent moment when that exact emotion was triggered. Write down any important details regarding the situation.**

   I'll provide a personal example. One of the dominant negative emotions I've felt throughout my life is panic, fortified by fear. And because of the extensive health-related challenges in the past, when the phone rang, it was often bad news from the doctor. So, these days, when my phone rings and it's a doctor's office calling, my stomach immediately drops even before I answer. As a trauma response, I freeze in anxiety . . . because history has proven it must be bad news. Below the surface of the panic is a subconscious learned belief. So, when that happens, I've learned to ask myself, *What does it mean if the doctor does call with a concern? What do I believe to be true about myself?* Historically, my answer was *It must mean that I am in trouble and that I am helpless, alone, abandoned, and destined for a disappointing life.*

And right there is the false identity, the belief that used to drive the dominant narrative of my life: *I am helpless and abandoned. I am a victim!*

3. **Ask yourself, *What does this mean for me when this scenario occurs?***

The presence of the dominant negative emotion you identified has less to do with the scenario itself and more with your core belief concerning your identity and safety in that or any other triggering situation. The negative emotion is simply an alarm, so pay attention. Arresting the *underlying belief* is crucial, because if we fail to address the lies, we empower them to dominate our lives. It's exactly why Paul implored us to "destroy arguments and every lofty opinion raised against the knowledge of God, and take every thought captive to obey Christ."[17]

That false belief is something you adopted through adverse circumstances. Circumstances indeed speak, but sadly, too many of us come to the wrong conclusions when fear is the dominant driver in our lives.

4. **Take that false identity or belief, whatever it is, to the Lord and ask Him, "When was the first time I learned and received [false identity/belief]?"**

So, using my example, I would ask the Lord, "When was the first time in my life I learned and believed that I was helpless and abandoned as a victim of life?" This step is important because that early memory—even though it may have occurred years ago—is stored like a picture on our cells all throughout the body. As such, it is still present to affect our physiology.[18] Of course, the ability for past memories to affect one's current reality extends to instances of trauma too. Bessel van der Kolk wrote, "When something reminds traumatized people of the past, their right brain reacts as if the traumatic event were happening in the present."[19] Thankfully, the One who knows us most intricately, who knit us together in our mothers' wombs,[20] will indeed search us and know us,[21] reveal to us issues of the heart not detectable by our own mind, and heal us. How great and *faithful* is our God!

5. **Now ask the Lord, "What do You say about [the memory/ experience]? What do You want me to know about who I am and who You are to me right now?"**

I'll never forget the first time I heard His answer, which was straight from Hebrews 13:5: "I will not in any way fail you nor give you up nor leave you without support. [I will] not, [I will] not, [I will] not in any degree leave you helpless nor forsake nor let [you] down (relax My hold on you)! [Assuredly not!]" (AMPC).

In that moment, the toxic thought and believed lie that I was inherently a victim of life, hopeless and helpless in my circumstances, was weakened. This is the power of knowing truth—the very truth that Jesus said would set us free.[22] Also, from the science of neuroplasticity, we know that replacing toxic thoughts with God's true thoughts about us will, over time, literally change the structure of our brains toward health and wholeness.

Going forward, it was my responsibility to bring *God's* eternal truth into the present reality anytime fear knocked on the door of my heart, even if it happened ten times a day. And in so doing, the soil of my heart received another level of healing, so that seeds of future potential and promise from the Lord had a readied rich bed on which to germinate and grow.

I encourage you to keep record of these guided sessions and include your mentor, pastor, or counselor in the deep work of processing through them and installing them in your daily life.

Wholeness, like any seed in soil, doesn't mature in a day; it matures *daily.* Commit to this process of checking *and working* the ground of your heart daily.

And above everything you do, with all your focus, think about what you're thinking about. Found your thoughts on the truth of the Word, which leads to life. Guard your mind from toxic thought patterns, pursue wholeness in your inner person, and protect the creative, emotional center of your life. After all, everything you are and everything you do start there. The quality of the soil will indeed determine the fruitfulness of the seed.

> Wholeness, like any seed in soil, doesn't mature in a day; it matures *daily.*

PERSONALIZE IT

THE POINT

Maturity should be the target of every believer, and each one of us should take responsibility for our health and growth. That's why we must regularly "work the ground" of our hearts.

THE PROMPT

Remember, information alone does not lead to transformation. Therefore, what is your specific plan to meet with a mentor to employ the self-awareness and guided exercise tools I provided in this chapter?

THE POSTURE

Once again, humility is a necessary posture from which to approach the transformation of our hearts. But I want to add hunger and a teachable spirit to the mix. This type of posture establishes the aim and focus of our minds and hearts away from independence and control and toward dependence on the presence of the Holy Spirit.

THE PRAYER

Father, I come to You in the name of Jesus. And by the power of the Holy Spirit, I ask You to search my heart. Know me. Examine me. Only You can change my heart. Not willpower. Not self-help. Not even clever ideas. It is only by Your Spirit that I am healed, restored, and transformed. So, as I apply the tools from this chapter, would You reveal anything that is hindering me from receiving the fullness of what You have for me? Give me a hearing ear to listen and respond to Your direction. Thank You, Lord. Amen.

ELEVEN

THE POWER OF A TRANSFORMED MIND

The ultimate freedom we have as human beings
is the power to select what we will allow or require
our minds to dwell upon.

—DALLAS WILLARD, *Renovation of the Heart*

Several years ago, I began working with a young man to unravel the narrative of fear and shame that had rendered him stuck in life, stemming back to his childhood. The tattered and coarsened ropes of believed lies that had been cinched around his heart decades prior still held him captive in isolation and fear, while his thoughts ran unrestrained in anticipation of the next inevitable disappointment. Though he appeared composed and sharp on the outside, it was clear that he was suffocating in defeat and despair on the inside, and I could not ignore his faint cry for help.

So, when we finally met, I knew we had to start from the beginning to uproot the underlying source of his pain and position him for the healing of his broken spirit. As we've learned, our earliest memories and experiences play a significant role in establishing the narrative from which we live life forward.

"These incessant, fearful thoughts . . ." I began. "What's your earliest memory of when they showed up in your mind?"

"Every night as a small child, as part of my bedtime routine," he explained, "I would beg my parents, 'Please don't go down-stairs. *Promise?*'"

Reluctantly, he went on to share that falling asleep without their assurance was nearly impossible. As he grew into adolescence, the mantra faded quickly, but the underlying root of fear did not. In fact, it matured. This held my attention, because his common childhood fears of the dark transposed into something quite insidious later in life. By his early twenties, a series of disappointing events and the accumulation of painful circumstances corroborated his motivation to create a life defined by self-protection and predictability. "Timid and clenched" is how he described his general temperament in those early days. Clearly, this was the fear of abandonment at work, and I wanted to see him get free . . . and *stay* free.

As our conversation ensued, he told me that every night after receiving his parents' promise to remain on the upstairs level of their house, he made sure to lock and double-check his bedroom windows, which, in his mind, prevented robbers and raccoons from entering his bedroom. With embarrassment veiled by a subtle smirk, he shared that the maniacal exercise extinguished any fear of being an unprotected, open target for assault, both emotionally and physically, during the night.

Attending to his story, I was shocked by his sensitivity at such a young age and amazed by the vividness of his descriptions, which were similar to those of actual robbing victims. So, curiously, I asked whether he or anyone in his family had ever been robbed or violated in the past.

"I don't think so," he replied. But that's precisely what fear and foreboding thoughts do: They create a "reality" based solely on speculation and untruth that's as real as if something tragic had actually happened.

And as for his imagery of robbers and raccoons? How ironic yet how specific. I reasoned that both represent prowlers that lurk in the night, which clarified another core fear deep in his soul: the fear of vulnerability and helplessness. As our time together evolved, he revealed that in addition to his parents' promise of staying nearby and the assurance of the windows being locked, his nightlight had to remain on. Though he was a very young boy at the time, only four or five years old, his childhood fear of the dark and of being left alone without protection translated into a full-blown, adult-sized fear of the unknown—which the life-and-death adversity he faced as a young adult then validated and exacerbated.

Gradually, and with a counselor's help, he came to recognize the common thread that ran through his childhood fears: the fear of losing control. I think that's the core fear for most of us, isn't it? This core fear (and the subsequent drive to take control of life) resulted from shame's successful leveraging of unhealed pain and ungrieved losses from his past.

Thus, shame wrote a new story and gave him a false identity. He received it because history created a precedent for how he viewed the world and what he learned to believe about himself. Shame told him he'd be safer if he isolated himself—that it was up to him to take care of himself and that doing so would let him avoid future losses. He was indeed stuck in the cycle of pain. This explained why, when we met, he was bound by a broken spirit, his hope atrophied by the ropes of fear, shame, and lies. And just as you've learned throughout this book, I believed his healing would be proportionate to the measure he surrendered his story to his Redeemer and engaged with the process of grieving his losses wholeheartedly. It would unfold as he forged a pathway to peace and allowed the Holy Spirit access to work the ground of his heart, extricating lies and replacing them with seeds of truth. This truth would not only set him free but also be a key player in his transformation, which would occur through the entire renewal of his mind.

So, as we concluded our time together, I told him, "The strength of our minds to steer our lives must not be underestimated." Without a doubt, the power of transformed thinking would be the focus of our next several sessions together. I must say that I grew to look forward to my time with him. And truth be told, it was easy to find that young man—because all I had to do was look in the mirror.

COMING TO THE WRONG CONCLUSIONS

Like the psalmist who asked, "Why are you cast down, O my soul, and why are you in turmoil within me?"[1] I regularly peered within the recesses of my soul in an effort to discover the root of the tormenting fear that fueled most of my anxious thoughts and mindsets. Of course, this work of "meeting" with myself was always done in the presence of my counselor, led by the Holy Spirit, and under the authority of Scripture.

Looking back, I've always had a meticulous and contemplative personality, which isn't inherently a bad thing. I'm extremely driven and detail-oriented, and precision is the name of my game. But overextended and under stress, "precise" becomes "anxious and controlling." In fact, growing up, I'm sure I could have been labeled as compulsive and neurotic. Everything had a place, and if something wasn't in its place, I felt as though *I* was out of place.

Well, as you know by now, fear took center stage in my heart as a child. But fast-forward a few decades, and I was up against the ropes once again as an adult. Because of the accumulation of painful life circumstances, fear and anxiety dominated my thought life in an unrelenting manner. Most of the time, my anxious meditations were completely irrational yet utterly debilitating, especially by late 2013 when the severe headaches began.

I had never experienced acute physical pain to this extent before. Out of the blue on a Wednesday night, I was nearly knocked off my feet by a sharp jolt in my left temple. Fifteen minutes later, I felt another stab. Thirty minutes later, I was flat on my back on the couch after three more painful jolts to the side of my head. The next day, I was symptom-free. Once Friday arrived, however, I got pummeled by another barrage of cluster headaches. This pattern continued for about a month, and in that span of time, do you think I sat quietly and waited for the storm to pass? Do you think I believed my doctor when he *assured* me they were cluster headaches? Not a chance. Instead, I ran my symptoms through Google, which only turned up the volume on the fearful thoughts racing through my mind and heightened the stress response in my body, creating even more uncomfortable physical symptoms. The narrative went like this:

> Your mom died of cancer + You have her DNA + *You* have cancer + You were diagnosed with MS when they found lesions on your brain + The MRI of your brain missed the tumor on the side of your brain + The doctor is wrong + Those lesions are actually tumors + The sharp pains are evidence of a tumor pressing on the side of your brain + You're dying = **My childhood fears were true all along.** I *was* abandoned. I am vulnerable and helpless. The unknown *must* be feared because it is always bad, and now my life is about to end, which proves that I *was* always "useless and stupid." But now, and even worse, I *am* obviously "worthless and forgettable."

Maybe for you, the equation looks more like this:

> Because the economy is unstable, I'm afraid of losing my job and all my clients + If I lose this job, I will not be able to find another one + I'm not as capable as I thought I was + My boss just shut his office door + He's talking about me + I *am* going to lose my job + I *will* lose my security + I *will* be ashamed because my security is in my job + I *will* be rejected by people I thought were my friends + I will be alone = **I am a failure**.

Let's get under the hood of these narratives for a moment to understand how they run freely in our minds. Both are reinforced by a perpetual cycle of accusation, speculation, and rumination, which you'll see on the next page.

The purpose of *accusation*, which emanates from the Enemy, is to unseat us from our belief and trust in our identity in Christ—

the foundation for living an overcoming, resilient life.[2] *Speculation* is when we form theories about the issues of life without having firm evidence to support our thoughts. This is the foundation of worry. And *rumination* is when we engage "in a repetitive negative thought process that loops continuously in the mind without end or completion."[3]

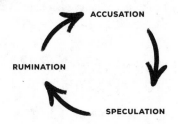

The cycle starts as follows:

The Enemy plants the seed of a thought through a lie and an **accusation**: "You are worthless and forgettable. Because you didn't manage your stress in the first place, there's no hope of getting out of this situation or out of this state of being. It's your fault."

With an unrenewed mind and a broken spirit, you allow that seed of thought to sit atop your conscious mind. You **speculate** that it might actually be true because of unsubstantiated, unrelated evidence in your life. Things like "What if this is the reason I'm sick and lonely?" and "What if something worse happens? Maybe my kids *are* in danger. Who will provide for them if I'm not here?" are constant considerations.

It isn't long before speculation becomes **rumination,** where "It might happen" becomes "It *will* happen," and your agreements with the Enemy's lies become your subconscious declarations: "Sickness is my lot in life. I am worthless. I am forgettable. It is my fault, and there's no hope out of this situation." And it is from those internal declarations that strongholds in the mind are built and you become a prisoner in a war you were designed to win.

Sadly, it doesn't stop there. Through your partnership with his initial lie, the Enemy takes advantage of the inroad to your mind and, with repeated accusations, fortifies the very stronghold keeping you captive.

When you don't take an accusation—a *thought*—captive and submit it to the Lord through His Word, you will spend your days trapped in anxiety-ridden rumination. This cycle will not only distract you from the truth that will set you free but also deplete you of the energy to get up, take courage, and follow the Lord in your purpose.

THE STRENGTH OF OUR MINDS
TO STEER OUR LIVES

In both scenarios, what is the result of these fear-driven, obsessive thought patterns? Like we pointed out in chapter 10, it is a false identity: a reproach that we receive as truth, even though it was founded on a lie! *This* is the power of a thought. In these specific cases, it is the power of a series of toxic thoughts left unchecked, aroused by a broken spirit. And *this* is why we must not underestimate the strength of our minds to steer our lives. Proverbs 15:15 illustrates this point, saying, "For the despondent, every day brings trouble; for the happy heart, life is a continual feast" (NLT).

In other words, the everyday lives of those who are depressed and lack hope are distressed *all the more* by anxious thoughts and fearful apprehension about the future. But those whose hearts are cheerful (remember that the heart includes the mind) enjoy a continual feast of the goodness of the Lord, even amid trying circumstances. Perhaps, then, the psalmist's invitation to "taste and see that the LORD is good!"[4] is more than a good idea. Perhaps it's a tangible opportunity to perceive *and experience* the goodness and favor of our Father in every season of life. This is the power of a fixed focus, for whatever we focus on flourishes.

THE MATURITY AND MOVEMENT OF THOUGHTS

You see, when validated by emotions, both toxic (destructive) and true (life-giving) thoughts become beliefs that compose our mindsets. And like eyeglass lenses, our mindsets calibrate the way we see ourselves and the world around us.

But it doesn't stop there. Our mindsets steer our actions, and in turn, our actions validate and fortify our mindsets and beliefs. Repeated actions become habits, and habits form character. And character most often drives us to live as either *stewards* of our purpose and "more than conquerors" or *victims* of unfair, unjust circumstances.

In the two narratives I shared, the facts were frightening. But the true circumstances didn't prevent the resulting untruths in each cycle of thought. Untruths like these will hijack our hope and hamper our ability to navigate life with stability and maturity as sons and daughters of a King who promised "I will never leave you nor forsake you."[5]

Are sickness and disease devastating? Yes, of course. Is losing a job embarrassing and frightening? Without a doubt. But neither experience substantiates the false identity (delivered as a fear-incited lie) of "I am worthless and forgettable" or "I am a failure." Because of our position in Christ,[6] our true identities have nothing to do with what befalls us in life. Yet pain and loss hopelessly attempt to challenge the validity of that truth, don't they? Therefore, we must refute the lies that seek to entrap us by confronting them with the truth of who we are and whose we are and regularly auditing our thought lives. If we don't, we will think, feel, and act as if those lies are true. As a result, we will unintentionally receive, empower, and *embody* the false identity in our everyday lives and in the context of all our relationships! This is the consequence of toxic thinking and an unrenewed mind.

Two well-respected psychiatrists expound on this notion from a neuroscientific perspective, describing "the process of how a deceptive brain message progresses to unhealthy behaviors and habits." According to the doctors' cycle, a "deceptive brain message" (a thought, urge, or desire) leads to "uncomfortable physical or emotional sensations" (such as cravings), which in turn leads to "habitual unhealthy responses." This relieves the distress momentarily—until the cycle repeats itself.[7] In no small fashion, this is precisely why no thought must be left unchecked before it leaves our conscious minds.

GUARD YOUR HEART = GUARD YOUR MIND

About the structure of a thought, Dr. Caroline Leaf, a renowned communication pathologist and neuroscientist, said, "Thoughts are real, physical things that occupy mental real estate. Moment by moment, every day, you are changing the structure of your brain through your thinking. When we hope, it is an activity of the mind that changes the structure of our brain in a positive and normal direction."[8] And thus, we're once again reminded of the preeminence of Solomon's admonition to "guard your heart above all else, for it determines the course of your life."[9]

The heart, as you will recall from the last couple of chapters, is not only the seat of emotions but also the inner part of one's being that includes the mind, thinking, reflection, and memory.[10] Therefore, we guard our hearts by taking thoughts captive and renewing our minds according to God's truth found in the Scriptures. How critical this is to understand, because our thoughts and emotions don't necessarily validate truth; they validate our *perceptions* of truth, which might be wrong! Therein lies a challenge: It is extremely difficult to discern eternal truth leading to freedom and life in our mental and emotional health (let alone our spiritual walk) when we have not developed the discipline of regularly establishing our focus on things that are good, true, and excellent,[11] especially first thing in the morning.[12]

> Our thoughts and emotions don't necessarily validate truth; they validate our *perceptions* of truth, which might be wrong!

Sadly, many people live distracted in front of screens for several hours each day, absorbing the trauma of a fractured, insecure, dysfunctional world and receiving messaging that vies not only for their attention but also for their buy-in. This reality foreshadows a broader implication regarding our thought life, of course. For when we pursue transformation in our thinking, we not only will live healthier lives from the inside out but also will be spiritually mature enough to offer solutions to a world that is desperate for help. The apostle Paul told us how to engage with this reality when he wrote, "Do not be conformed to this world, but be transformed by the renewal of your mind, that by testing you may discern what is the will of God, what is good and acceptable and perfect."[13]

As we renew our minds, therefore, our ability to think, feel, and choose[14] *according to truth* will result in self-directed neuroplastic adaptation—changing the physical structures of the brain[15]—and will thereby alter the brain's automatic stress response, which directly affects our physiology. A recurring verse in this book exemplifies the consequences of this reality: "A calm and undisturbed mind and heart are the life and health of the body, but envy, jealousy, and wrath are like rottenness of the bones."[16]

Clearly, our thoughts affect our physiology in a powerful way. But how? Leaf explained:

> As you think, your thoughts are activated, which in turn activates your attitude, because your attitude is all of your thoughts put together and reflects your state of mind. This attitude is reflected in the chemical secretions that are released. Positive attitudes cause the secretion of the correct amount of chemicals, and negative attitudes distort the chemical secretions in a way that disrupts their natural flow. The chemicals are like little cellular signals that translate the information of your thought into a physical reality in your body and mind, creating an emotion. The combination of thoughts, emotions, and resulting attitudes, impacts your body in a positive or negative way.[17]

Simply stated, as we change our thoughts, we will adjust our attitudes and mindsets, which will alter our biochemistry and eventually change our lives! But how do we accomplish this? How do we effect meaningful change in our mental and emotional health? The apostle Paul provides a brilliant prescription for doing so in 2 Corinthians 10:4–5: "The weapons of our warfare are not of the flesh but have divine power to destroy strongholds. We destroy arguments and every lofty opinion raised against the knowledge of God, and take every thought captive to obey Christ."

Did you catch that? We *destroy arguments* that take place on the battlefield of the mind by taking our thoughts—not just negative thoughts but *every* thought—captive to obey Christ. Hence, we must heed the wisdom of the late Dallas Willard, who said, "As we first turned away from God in our thoughts, so it is in our thoughts that the first movements toward the renovation of the heart occur. Thoughts are the place where we can and must begin to change."[18]

GET UNDER THE HOOD

Because thoughts that establish our mindsets are the framework for the stories we tell ourselves, I want to get under the hood of the narratives that orient much of the way we view our lives, past, present, and future. One key factor influencing these narratives is how we remember our life experiences. *How* we remember is as important as *what* we remember and is largely shaped by *who* we believe we are. So, we must ask ourselves, while our memories and lived experiences are always real, are our perspectives and conclusions about them always accurate and consistent? Or do our default narratives about who we believe we are, both in and of ourselves and in relation to the world around us, color them?

Bessel van der Kolk shed some light on the subject: "Such autobiographical memories are not precise reflections of reality; they are stories we tell to convey our personal take on our experience."[19] I believe that our personal takes on our experiences are indeed shaped by either the security that comes from knowing our true identity in Christ or the insecurity that is born from a broken spirit. And thus the point: We don't see the world as it is; we see the world *as we are* (or as we *believe* we are).

Now, as a primer to what I'm about to share, in no way do I want to approach this subject in a reductionistic manner that lacks sensitivity to the uniqueness of your lived experiences. Please don't misinterpret my angle. However, I do believe there are two prominent archetypes that best describe us *as we are* in the myriad of challenges and triumphs we face: the victim and the overcomer. These archetypes shape not only the way we remember our past but also how we see life in the present and into the future.

Archetype #1: The Victim

The victim's outlook on life is brought into focus by hopelessness, resentment, helplessness, defeat, and despair due to the pervading presence of a broken spirit. Their thought life is consumed by negative, toxic, anxiety-ridden rumination. Shame drives the fundamental narrative of their life. Self-protection and self-promotion by way of insecurity is their familiar and reflexive posture. And in such cases, they bring the past into the present, where open and unhealed soul wounds hemorrhage on their everyday life and into their relationships.

Sadly, victims' seasons become their stories, and their stories, their identities. They arrive at the conclusion "This is who I am" after loss or disappointment—a core wounded belief that for them is indistinguishable from "This is what happened to me." Thus, Willard's words bear repeating: "Thoughts are the place where we can and must begin to change."[20]

That said, I want to make a clear distinction. When I describe the victim archetype, I am talking specifically (and only) about when our adversities and losses become our *identity* and when toxic, unrenewed thinking becomes our status quo. I know this to be true because "victim" was my reality and my identity (a false identity at that) for a season of my life.

Not one of us has escaped adversity and loss in this life. We live in a fallen world awaiting redemption. It's just that suffering loss *in* life (an unavoidable reality) isn't synonymous with being a victim *of* life.

Archetype #2: The Overcomer

On the other hand, overcomers are those whose lives have been marked by adversity, who bear the scars of loss in their past, but whose scars tell a story of hope and healing. The affections of their hearts are anchored in a superior reality: the kingdom of God, whose King redeems and restores as an innate quality of His nature. In fact, they have surrendered their stories to a King whose name is "Redeemer," and they have made Him the Lord over their inner lives. Overcomers realize the priority of continually renewing their minds in the truth of the Scriptures, where, by the power of the Holy Spirit, they will be transformed from the inside out. They are not shy about the pain of their past, for they know that true faith does not require them to deny a problem's existence. Instead, faith refuses their problems the opportunity to unseat their trust and confidence in the power, wisdom, and goodness of the Lord.

Not only that, but overcomers understand that faith is not the state of having certainty about outcomes; instead, genuine faith requires us to embrace mystery *with trust* as part of our journeys through life, just as we discussed in chapter 7. Moreover, hope, the joyful expectation of good,[21] is the sure and steadfast anchor of their souls.[22] Because of that, the adversities and challenges that have befallen them are not indicative of their true identity[23] as "more than conquerors" in all things.

THE LINCHPIN OF TRANSFORMATION

After framing up the archetypes of victim and overcomer, do you better understand that *how* we see is informed by motivations of either fear, where the broken spirit thrives, or perfect love—in which we face trials of many kinds not with doubt, despair, and distrust but with steadfastness, hope, and faith?

Reinforcing the central theme of this book, healing the broken spirit is a linchpin issue for transformation and wholeness. The broken spirit views life through trauma, innate defeat, and hopelessness, which is the environment where destructive patterns of thinking thrive. This is why eliminating toxic thinking patterns and broken narratives of fear, shame, and dysfunction is a nonnegotiable factor to our well-being.

A WORD ABOUT TRAUMA AND TRAUMATIC MEMORIES

Having said that, I cannot ignore the fact that for many people (maybe *you*), some memories that flood their hearts and minds are not simply difficult but traumatic. And these memories are stored not just in the brain but also in cells all over the body.[24] So, though the focus of this chapter is renewing our minds, if trauma of any kind has been part of your story as it was for me, I want to first acknowledge your pain with the utmost compassion. I strongly advise you to seek out a licensed professional Christian counselor who specializes in trauma therapy and can lead you through treatment that includes regular counseling sessions as well as inner healing prayer. In my own healing journey, emotional freedom techniques (EFT) and eye movement desensitization and reprocessing (EMDR) have been remarkably helpful.

Therefore, if you have experienced (or are experiencing) trauma in your life, please take your time and take care with the help of a skilled Christian counselor and a trusted mental health professional. Trauma must not be ignored, but it does not have to run the rest of your life.

Let's continue to explore the power of a transformed mind through a case study provided to us in 1 Samuel 30.

STRENGTHENING OURSELVES IN THE LORD

Just before I teach you my four-step method to renew your mind on a regular basis, I want to illustrate why we must not underestimate the strength of our minds to steer our lives. Along with that principle, I want you to see the way an "overcomer" identity will not only shape how we view our life experiences but also ground us in emotional stability and provide a strategy for personal, internal victory when chaos arises all around us.

Enter David. By the time we meet up with him in 1 Samuel 30, David had risen to power as a general in Saul's army. He was winning not only victories in battle but also notoriety among the people.[25] But his success became a snare to Saul, whose jealousy raged to the point that he began a hunt to kill David. And despite two opportunities David had to kill Saul, his integrity and trust in the ways of the Lord motivated him to spare Saul's life.[26]

Well, when we pick up the scene in chapter 30, David's camp in the city of Ziklag had been pillaged. Forget the fact that people used to sing his praises to the tune of "Saul has struck down his thousands, and David his ten thousands."[27] The women and children of Ziklag had been taken captive, and David's men were mad. In fact, they wanted David dead too. Yet what was David's posture? From whom did he receive his identity? And what was the subsequent narrative running through David's mind? While Scripture doesn't explicitly reveal this information, we do know that he didn't run away from the distress in his soul or allow it to unseat his focus and dictate his choices.[28] Instead, he strengthened himself in the Lord and then inquired of Him, which provided the emotional stability, spiritual stamina, and rational strategy to win the battle and recover all that had been lost. How did he accomplish this? I believe it was by recounting the faithfulness of the Lord to lead him into victory in the past.

You see, a person whose heart is steadfast and whose focus is fixed on a greater reality than the seemingly insurmountable obstacles in their way can say with confidence, like David, "Though an army encamp against me, *my heart shall not fear; though war arise against me, yet I will be confident.* One thing have I asked of the LORD, that will I seek after: that I may dwell in the house of the LORD all the days of my life, to gaze upon the beauty of the LORD and to inquire in his temple. For *he will hide me in his shelter* in the day of trouble; he will conceal me under the cover of his tent; he will lift me high upon a rock."[29]

What an example for us to follow. Any battle we face on the

outside must first be won on the inside, for the battleground is indeed the mind. That's precisely why I developed the SEED Method in the heat of my own battles. Because if we don't manage our inner world, it will eventually manage us.

> Any battle we face on the outside must first be won on the inside, for the battleground is indeed the mind.

THE SEED METHOD FOR RENEWING YOUR MIND

The SEED Method is my four-step strategy for renewing the mind, based on principles of neuroscience and the Scriptures. And because thoughts are like seeds that fall on the soil of the heart (read: mind), the following four steps create the acronym *SEED*. The goal of this exercise is to help you audit your thought life more effectively so that anxious, destructive thoughts are secured ("taken captive" to use Paul's language), examined, exposed to, and replaced with truth *before* they become rooted beliefs, mindsets, and narratives that run your life. (I hope you'll notice similarities between this exercise and the guided exercise from chapter 10.)

Dr. Caroline Leaf said, "To make changes in our thoughts and subsequent communication, we need to be strategic, proactive and deliberate about our thinking. We need to try to be aware of what we are thinking about every day."[30] This practice, which scientists call "metacognition,"[31] is indeed the heartbeat of the SEED Method. For when we secure our thoughts, examine their origin, expose them to truth, and decide to redirect our thoughts in accordance with truth, we position ourselves for transformation by the renewal of our minds, just as Paul wrote in Romans 12:2.

As we begin, I recommend that you always journal your thoughts and subsequent findings while practicing the SEED Method. Studies have shown that writing expressively about your worries on paper offloads them and frees up mental space to see them objectively, which allows you to be more focused and less reactive.[32]

Step One: Secure

Step one is to *secure* a dominant anxious thought in the forefront of your mind so that you can think about your thinking. Maintain conscious awareness of the thought as if you were holding it like a physical object in your hands.[33] For example, last summer I was ruminating with anxiety about a medical test for which I was awaiting results. My specific thought was something like *I can't shake the feeling that I'm going to get bad news about my health.*

Step Two: Examine

The next step is to *examine* the motivating factors of that specific thought with the leading of the Holy Spirit. This is an effort to trace the breadcrumbs of the anxious thought and discover and diagnose the root of any believed lie that is keeping the underlying fear response alive. Let's go back to our working example, "I can't shake the feeling that I'm going to get bad news about my health."

Utilizing the SEED Method in this exact situation, I asked myself, *Despite what I feel right now, what did the doctor* actually *tell me when I was in his office?* Thinking objectively interrupted the cycle of anxious rumination and refocused my thoughts on the facts of what took place. What I remembered the doctor saying was "This blood test is routine for a person your age. You have nothing to worry about."

I then asked the Lord, "Will You show me why I am worried? What was the inciting incident that's dialing up the foreboding fear in my mind?" He reminded me that from childhood into my young adult years, most of the time my mom received a phone call from her oncologist, it was bad news. My regular exposure to those situations conditioned my soul to expect bad news from *any* doctor, even in my own life and under totally different circumstances. That of course is a trauma response.

Examining the thought further, I asked the Lord, "I know what the doctor said. But I'm still scared. What do You want me to know about this situation? And is there a lie that I'm believing?"

He responded, "Because of the accumulation of painful circumstances and losses in your life, you have come to the wrong conclusions about who you are because of what happened to you. Your anxious rumination is an indication that you believe you are alone in this. You believe *I* have forgotten about you. The lie you're believing is that your mom's fate is your fate, that her story is your story, and that her death was your fault. And because you have believed that lie, you're stuck in this vicious cycle of foreboding fear."

Bomb drop. The Lord not only answered my question but also revealed the inciting condition of my heart I could not have seen myself. And *that's* the point I want you to remember: The act of transformation involves not merely changing our minds but also revealing our core motivations and mindsets so that when our hearts are revealed, we can be healed. This is precisely what step two of the SEED Method is all about. Everything we do and everything we are come from an issue of the heart.

> The act of transformation involves not merely changing our minds but also revealing our core motivations and mindsets so that when our hearts are revealed, we can be healed.

Of equal importance to remember is that even though *you* will ask Him questions about your life, *you* aren't going to do the searching. Outside His help, you can't see what you need to see. Instead, the Holy Spirit, *the Spirit of Truth,* will not only search your heart but also lead and guide you into the truth about the condition of your heart. And that truth, when received and acted on, will set you free.[34] This is an important distinction to understand compared with the advice given to us by pop psychology and the self-help industry.

While secular humanism and many modern self-help strategies

encourage introspection and the discovery of "truth" within ourselves, I believe that advice is futile (let alone discouraging and
unwise) for our help comes from the Lord.[35] The Holy Spirit's job
is to search our hearts and try our anxious thoughts. This was
David's prayer in Psalm 139:23–24: "Search me, O God, and
know my heart! Try me and know my thoughts! And see if there
be any grievous way in me, and lead me in the way everlasting!"
By faith, we trust and believe that as the Holy Spirit searches us,
He will illuminate issues (believed lies, memories, situations, interactions, and conversations) that need to be dealt with in the
light of His presence.

But we can't stop there. It's one thing to uncover a lie, but that
lie must be replaced with truth. In fact, that's the point of step
three in the SEED Method.

Step Three: Expose

Though "I can't shake the feeling that I'm going to get bad news
about my health" was an understandable response to complex
post-traumatic stress, my anxious ruminations and foreboding
dread stemmed from a deeply implanted lie I had believed about
my life: My mom's fate was my fate and her story was my story.
And as a result of receiving and believing that lie, I unintentionally empowered it to mature in my soul and spirit.

Thus, I would like to suggest that one of the greatest tools in
the Enemy's arsenal against you is deception. In fact, Jesus said
that lies are the Enemy's "native language."[36] And if he can bait
you to believe a lie that then is sown as a seed in the soil of your
heart and remains unaddressed, you will think and act as though
it is truth. This of course demonstrates what happens when perfect love—which drives out every trace of fear[37]—is not abound-
ing in our hearts. In such cases, fear thrives and introduces torment
in our souls.

So, examining your anxious thoughts in the Lord's presence
allows you to locate the source of a thought. It reveals the core

believed lie that was empowered to thrive in your life. But *exposing* that thought (and the attached lie) to truth will uproot its influence from your thought life, as well as overthrow and destroy the strongholds it has built.[38] How is this accomplished? And how do we combat lies? With Scripture.

So, I asked myself, *What does the Word say about my situation?* and *How does Scripture confront my faulty belief that my fate is sealed and that my life is worthless?* Let's look at some of my findings:

Blessed be the Lord, Who bears our burdens and carries us day by day, even the God Who is our salvation! (Psalm 68:19, AMPC)

Because he holds fast to me in love, I will deliver him;
    I will protect him, because he knows my name.
When he calls to me, I will answer him;
    I will be with him in trouble;
    I will rescue him and honor him.
With long life I will satisfy him
    and show him my salvation. (Psalm 91:14–16)

Lean on, trust in, and be confident in the Lord with all your heart and mind and do not rely on your own insight or understanding. In all your ways know, recognize, and acknowledge Him, and He will direct and make straight and plain your paths. (Proverbs 3:5–6, AMPC)

Surely he has borne our griefs
    and carried our sorrows;
yet we esteemed him stricken,
    smitten by God, and afflicted.
But he was pierced for our transgressions;
    he was crushed for our iniquities;
upon him was the chastisement that brought us peace,
    and with his wounds we are healed. (Isaiah 53:4–5)

I will ask the Father, and He will give you another Comforter (Counselor, Helper, Intercessor, Advocate, Strengthener, and Standby), that He may remain with you forever—The Spirit of Truth, Whom the world cannot receive (welcome, take to its heart), because it does not see Him or know and recognize Him. But you know and recognize Him, for He lives with you [constantly] and will be in you. I will not leave you as orphans [comfortless, desolate, bereaved, forlorn, helpless]; I will come [back] to you. (John 14:16–18, AMPC)

There is no fear in love; but perfect love casts out fear, because fear involves torment. But he who fears has not been made perfect in love. (1 John 4:18, NKJV)

I want you to remember that this step in the SEED Method isn't about disclaiming the facts of what you're feeling and thinking. Instead, it involves aiming your heart at a superior reality amid your anxiety. In other words, it's not denying your anxiety; it's denying your anxiety license to control your everyday life.

So, after having exposed my anxious thought to the truth of the Word, a *decision* (an action) must follow. That is the fourth and final step in the SEED Method.

Step Four: Decide

What comes out of step three is valuable information. But information alone will not change our lives. Instead, when we consistently apply the information we gain, we're on the road to transformation. So, for this step, I highly recommend that you have a stack of blank index cards on hand.

Pick one of the scriptures from your time of examination and write it out on one side of the card. Let's say you choose Psalm 68:19 (AMPC) from the verses given above. After writing it on the card, I want you to use either the other side of the card or the space just below the verse to make that scripture personal. For instance, you might write something like "Blessed be the Lord,

Who bears *my* burdens and carries *me* day by day, even the God Who is *my* salvation." Then, keep the card with you all day. I got in the habit of placing mine on my dashboard so that I could carefully glance at it as I drove. Not only that, but I would also speak my personalized belief statement out loud.

This is indeed the process of *deciding* what we will focus on. And just in case I haven't said it enough throughout the book, I'll say it one more time: *Whatever we focus on flourishes.* In fact, this part of the exercise is exactly what Solomon wrote in Proverbs 4:20–23: "My son, *attend to my words;* consent and submit to my sayings. Let them not depart from your sight; *keep them in the center of your heart.* For they are life to those who find them, healing and health to all their flesh. Keep and guard your heart with all vigilance and above all that you guard, for out of it flow the springs of life" (AMPC).

Let's quickly recap the SEED Method:

Secure your thought so that you are consciously aware of it.

Examine the motivating factors of that specific thought with the leading of the Holy Spirit.

Expose that thought (and the attached lie) to truth, which will uproot its influence from your mind. How is this accomplished? With Scripture.

Decide to consistently place your focus on the truth of the Word, which will begin the process of installing a new thought in your mind. The Word of God, by the Holy Spirit, contains the power to change your life from the inside out.

RENEWAL OF THE MIND ISN'T A ONETIME EVENT

Considering the SEED Method and all the additional advice and scientific research regarding the power of our thought lives, why do many of us keep coming back to base camp on the issue of managing our inner lives? Why are we sidelined by toxic thinking? Is it because we hear the advice but don't really listen to it? Maybe. Is it that we do listen but don't know how to apply it? Perhaps. But let me propose another idea: Many of us do hear and apply sound wisdom about the strength of our thoughts. However, we've turned scriptures into fortune-cookie slogans without pursuing the Spirit who gives life to the very words we read. And when that doesn't work, we write the whole thing off and return to the world's self-preservation, self-creation, willpower-driven self-help tactics, not to mention our old habits.

Moreover, I believe we get stuck because we don't pursue the continual renewing of the mind. We don't set our minds and keep them set. And then when we don't see the results we want, we try harder. So while we might be able to change our minds about some things, our best efforts (whether by willpower or intention) aren't enough to change our mindsets long-term.

Store shelves are chock-full of books (many of which are far more scientific than this one) about mindsets and the power of our thoughts. But the wrestle I'm in continues to make me wonder, *If the influx of new books is outpacing the change people are experiencing, where is the disconnect?* Why aren't people experiencing lasting change? Why do we keep reverting to old habits and dumpster-fire thinking patterns that ultimately keep us smooth sailing down a path toward mediocre living?

Well, I think we can trace the answer back to our working thesis: Transforming hearts and healing broken spirits beat behavior modification all day long. And heart transformation requires repetition over time with specific focus, through surrender to a power that is not of our own creation. But it doesn't end there.

THE POWER OF A TRANSFORMED MIND

The roadmap to wholeness is not just about getting out of a ditch. It's about getting on the path to transformation. In any of the examples we've talked about thus far, know this: The Lord isn't merely interested in healing us. His eternal purposes for us as His delegated authorities here on the earth require a deeper work that leads to wholeness in our spirits, souls, and bodies.

He wants us to experience total and constant renewal in the spirit of our minds so that we taste and see His goodness, anchor the affections of our hearts to His kingdom values, and access supernatural resources in our everyday lives to see His kingdom expand. As we do so, He wants the fruit of our transformation to be a great sign to those who are far from Him. This was the case for heroes of the faith like Joshua, Caleb, Joseph, Esther, and Daniel.

God has always desired sonship for us. Scripture says that Jesus was "the firstborn among many brethren."[39] The *many brethren* is talking about us. And with that great privilege comes a call to pursue transformation from the inside out, by the Holy Spirit's power in our lives, and to answer one critical question: "Who do you think you are?"

PERSONALIZE IT

THE POINT

We must never underestimate the strength of our minds to steer our lives.

THE PROMPT

Because our thoughts and emotions validate our *perceptions* of truth, not necessarily truth itself, what specific steps will you take today to renew your mind by the power of the Holy Spirit and the authority of the Scriptures? How will you develop the reflexive skill to take *every* thought captive and lead it to obey Christ? The SEED Method is a useful tool for this.

THE POSTURE

Any battle we face on the outside must first be won on the inside, for the battleground is indeed the mind. That's why we must learn how to strengthen ourselves in the Lord on a regular basis, let alone prioritize the continual renewing of our minds.

THE PRAYER

Father, as I pursue the continual renewing of my mind, I thank You that the Spirit of Truth, Your Holy Spirit, will lead and guide me into all truth. Truth sets me free, Lord, and I want to walk in freedom from lies, bitterness, resentment, indignation, ungrieved losses, and unresolved disappointment, as well as everything that is false and any other soul condition that would hinder me from walking uprightly in maturity and wholeness. I want to represent You well in this life, and I desire to think, feel, and act according to Your ways. It's in Jesus's name that I pray these things. Amen.

PART III

THE BECKONING

TWELVE

WHO DO YOU THINK YOU ARE?

There is no question that the journey of finding our truly
authentic self in Christ and rooting our identity in this
reality is dramatically different from the agenda of
self-fulfillment promoted by pop psychology.

—DAVID G. BENNER, *The Gift of Being Yourself*

Being a rather shy and private person, I was at first taken aback
when, two minutes after sitting down for coffee together for the
first time in months and with barely enough time for me to re-
move my winter coat, my longtime friend and mentor asked,
"Christopher, who do you think you are?"

I'm not sure why his question caught me off guard, but nonetheless, I didn't like the surprising feeling of intimidation moments after we said hello. Add to that, beginning our meeting this
way made me rather nervous (and maybe irritated), because I
wasn't really interested in rehashing my whole story, even though
I had sought his counsel for years. Enough of my "Groundhog
Day." I was exhausted, was in pain, and just wanted to catch up
and talk, which is why I thought meeting with an old mentor-
friend might help. Maybe I had been wrong.

At his question, I may have rolled my eyes and thought to myself, *I'm in no mood for this.* As I felt the tension in my chest mount
and a storm of shame and defensiveness begin brewing inside me,
sweat began to form on my palms. I looked down at the floor and

sheepishly replied, "I . . . I . . . I mean, I'm . . ." I paused for what felt like minutes. "I'm hurting and I just want help, okay?" I answered, barely above a whisper, lifting my gaze away from the coffee-stained oak tabletop toward him.

Tears began to well up in my eyes. Cloaked in his familiar posture of compassion that had earned my trust so many years ago, he set his cup of coffee down and leaned in. "I know you're hurting. And I *am* here to help," he said. "But, Christopher, 'hurting' isn't who you are; it's *how* you are." He was right, but I didn't want anything to do with it. "Who are you today?" he pressed.

I shuddered. "I don't know. I can't see it. At least not today. All I see is brokenness. That's all everyone else sees too. I mean, I used to be—"

"The one who always wore a smile, who never lived life absent of hope?" he interrupted.

"Yeah, you got me," I conceded as tears flowed freely down my wearied countenance. He didn't have to say another word for his gentle probing to continue straight into my heart. "What are you getting at?" I pressed.

"Stay with me," he said. I could tell he was about to make his point. "Two of the most important questions we must answer in life are whether we believe God is fully who He says He is . . ." He paused, as if to lock his eyes even more intently on me. "And whether we believe *we are* who He says we are, especially when we face crisis, loss, or any significant obstacle that challenges our sense of safety and belonging. Christopher, you know this, but you're in a critical spot right now, so I want to emphasize a point. Who you believe you are and *whose* you believe you are is not about aligning your mind with a simple fact. I mean, that's *part* of it. But the greater point of knowing requires experience—history with the Lord, if you will. It requires engaging your heart, even when it has been broken into a thousand pieces. It's a reality, a *conviction,* from which you orient yourself in everyday life, right in the middle of your own chaos. And that's the challenge for a lot of people, because crisis, loss, disappointment, betrayal, sickness, and unrelenting fear, things like that, are loud, sometimes louder than the still, small voice of the Lord, right? They clamor for our attention."

"And our focus," I quickly added.

"Exactly," he said. "And this is why settling the issue of our identity in truth—*in Christ*—is like building a house on—"

"The rock," I interjected.

"Yes, precisely," he confirmed. "And that's why I asked you the question 'Who do you think you are?' It's not to ignore what you're walking through right now. But it is to fortify you from the inside out *as* you walk through this valley. It's to shore up the foundation of the house called 'your life' on stability and truth.

"You know, for some people, especially when they have been through a lot, like you, when their spirit has been broken and they're stuck in life after loss, deciphering truth from their true experiences is a challenge. And so, when asked that simple question, they interpret it as a shame-filled taunt, like *Who do you think you are to believe you're going to get well at this point in time? It's too late.* And that's just how the Enemy works, isn't it? His voice is accusatory and condemning, and the traces of his handiwork lead to shame and isolation. On the other hand, however, when the Holy Spirit asks the same question, it's never a taunt. Instead, it's an invitation to 'look up' with the eyes of your heart to your Helper and, as you've passionately told me in times past, to take courage and get up from everything that has held you down and to respond to His call to transformation in your true identity.

"Knowing who you are and *whose* you are," he continued, "is a foundation stone for healing. Build on that."

CLOAKED IN SHAME AND A FALSE IDENTITY

Now, years separated from that hinge moment in my healing journey, I'm convinced all the more about a critical factor in this work of transformation: the preeminent need for healing a broken spirit. Like we have discussed, when our spirits are broken, when we're stuck in cycles of pain and overcome by the vices of shame, we won't readily take courage or get up. Rather, we'll *take cover and stay down* because life's adversities and losses have validated our broken, faulty belief that we have been rejected, abandoned, and left to take care of ourselves. And like we discussed in the last chapter, when we live according to an untruth, we empower it to thrive in our lives. Sadly, this is the story for many believers today.

Self-protected and isolated, hedged in by broken spirits and crippled by the weight of ungrieved losses and unresolved disappointments, many tragically forge a new way of living, cloaked in a reproach of shame that expresses itself through a false identity. As you'll remember from earlier in the book, the strength of shame is that it hooks itself to our identity and recalibrates the way we see *everything*. This is the modus operandi of the false self, of which a medical doctor wrote, "The false self plays its deceptive role, ostensibly protecting us but doing so in a way that is programmed to keep us fearful—of being abandoned, losing support, not being able to cope on our own, not being able to *be* alone."[1]

To offset this soul state, therefore, those who live from the false self overextend and exhaust themselves in relationships and activities that are not based on desire or even a sense of calling. Instead, they live from a motivation of people-pleasing and insecurity, from "the fear of not living up to others' expectations."[2] Affirmation and applause become their drugs of choice to compensate for their unfamiliarity with the inexhaustible joy and sense of fulfillment that come through sonship, not through good performance.[3]

But why do so many settle for such a way of life? While the answer to this is found within the nuances of each one's personal history, I propose that many have settled for such a diminished way of living from the false self for so long that they would not recognize everyday life any other way.

Brennan Manning, author of *Abba's Child*, answered the same question this way:

First, because repressed memories from childhood that laid the pattern for self-deception are too painful to recall and thus remain carefully concealed. Faint voices from the past stir vague feelings of angry correction and implied abandonment. . . .

The second reason the imposter settles for less life is plain old cowardice. As a little one, I could justifiably cop a plea and claim that I was powerless and defenseless. But in the autumn of my life, strengthened by so much love and affection and seasoned by endless affirmation, I must painfully acknowledge that I still operate out of a fear-based center.[4]

It is this exact fear motivation, exacerbated by shame's insidious activity, that substantiates the false identity birthed by the broken spirit. And as we've already learned, the presence of a broken spirit impedes the process of life transformation and thus halts healing and restoration. In these individuals' state of dilapidation, brokenness is not simply what happened, they contend; "broken" is who they are. It is an issue of identity in which sufficiency in life is unfortunately found in one's deficiencies.

But God.

How gracious is the invitation of the Father toward us! It comes right in the middle of our greatest pain, when we have burrowed ourselves in hiddenness and isolation even from *Him*. And while we are crippled in heart and spirit by ungrieved losses and past disappointments, we are summoned *by name* to feast at the King's table, though we are yet bruised, timid, and limping. This is the testimony of Mephibosheth.

FROM DESOLATION TO SITTING AT THE KING'S TABLE

At the beginning of 2 Samuel, news had begun to spread about the deaths of Jonathan and his father, King Saul, and David was anointed king. Because it was customary for new kings to kill all remaining members of the former dynasty, Jonathan's five-year-old son, Mephibosheth, heir apparent to the throne as the son of Saul's firstborn, had reason to be afraid. Out of fear, as 2 Samuel

4:4 notes, Mephibosheth's nurse "took him up and fled, and as she fled in her haste, he fell and became lame."

Fast-forward to 2 Samuel 9. David, acting in a spirit opposite of revenge and self-protection despite Saul having made himself an enemy of David,[5] asked a former servant of Saul, "Is there not still someone of the house of Saul, that I may show the kindness of God to him?" Ziba, the servant, replied, "There is still a son of Jonathan; he is crippled in his feet."[6]

Let's go right to the Scriptures to see how the rest of the story played out. Second Samuel 9:4–13 says:

> The king said to him, "Where is he?" And Ziba said to the king, "He is in the house of Machir the son of Ammiel, at Lo-debar." Then King David sent and brought him from the house of Machir the son of Ammiel, at Lo-debar. And Mephibosheth the son of Jonathan, son of Saul, came to David and fell on his face and paid homage. And David said, "Mephibosheth!" And he answered, "Behold, I am your servant." And David said to him, "Do not fear, for I will show you kindness for the sake of your father Jonathan, and I will restore to you all the land of Saul your father, and you shall eat at my table always." And he paid homage and said, "What is your servant, that you should show regard for a dead dog such as I?"
>
> Then the king called Ziba, Saul's servant, and said to him, "All that belonged to Saul and to all his house I have given to your master's grandson. And you and your sons and your servants shall till the land for him and shall bring in the produce, that your master's grandson may have bread to eat. But Mephibosheth your master's grandson shall always eat at my table." Now Ziba had fifteen sons and twenty servants. Then Ziba said to the king, "According to all that my lord the king commands his servant, so will your servant do." So Mephibosheth ate at David's table, like one of the king's sons. And Mephibosheth had a young son, whose name was Mica. And all who lived in Ziba's house became

Mephibosheth's servants. So Mephibosheth lived in Jerusalem, for he ate always at the king's table. Now he was lame in both his feet.

This is a stunning picture of covenant-keeping, steadfast love. David, whose bond with Jonathan was once strong and enduring, sought out Mephibosheth, though the young man was crippled and in hiding. And from his place of desolation, even while he was lame, Mephibosheth was restored and brought to the king's table to dine *just like one of the king's sons.*

David didn't have to do this. Saul was dead. Jonathan was too. But this is how covenant love responds to life. Without question, it is opulent, abundant, and unfailing. Tears well in my eyes as I write these words because you and I are Mephibosheth. This is our story too. Because of His steadfast love for us, the Father calls us out of hiding, out of our own "Lo-debar," out of our shame-filled false identities, *even while we are yet lame and broken in spirit,* to dine at the King's table. Our seated place has been secured forever because of the finished work of King Jesus.

> Because of His steadfast love for us, the Father calls us out of hiding, out of our own "Lo-debar," out of our shame-filled false identities, *even while we are yet lame and broken in spirit,* to dine at the King's table.

Charles Spurgeon expounded on this thought: "The Lord's people are dear for another's sake. Such is the love which the Father bears to His only begotten, that for His sake He raises His lowly brethren from poverty and banishment, to courtly companionship, noble rank, and royal provision. Their deformity shall not rob them of their privileges. Lameness is no bar to sonship."[7]

Lameness is no bar to sonship. Read it again and receive it in your spirit: lameness is no bar to sonship. He calls you today. He beckons you to receive the true identity He has always had for you from the foundation of the earth: son, daughter, beloved . . . *Ab-*

ba's child. But you must answer the call. You must come out of hiding. You must take courage and get up by faith to receive what He has prepared for you: restoration, hope, and healing from the sting of death and loss from the seasons that cannot be erased from your life's story.

With a strong hand and an outstretched arm, the enduring love of the Father reaches for you today *in your broken state* and draws you to Himself! You need not hide your scars or your lameness at the King's table. Mephibosheth could not erase the fact that his father died at the hands of the Philistine army and that after being mortally wounded, his grandfather, King Saul, fell on his own sword and died. Nor could he erase the fact that as a young boy, he was dropped and became crippled. But for Mephibosheth, healing and restoration meant that he no longer needed to hide in fear and desolation even in the face of the scars from his past. Not only did he recover the land of his lineage, but he would also forever eat at the King's table—not as a "dead dog"[8] but as a son.

Though he experienced brokenness, "broken" was no longer his identity. This is the inherent strength of knowing our true identity in the face of disappointment and on the journey of transformation to heal what cannot be erased from our stories.

RECEIVING YOUR TRUE IDENTITY

Receiving our true identity is the fruit of abiding, not striving. David G. Benner said, "We do not find our true self by seeking it. Rather, we find it by seeking God."[9] That's exactly the point. It comes from the overflow of intimacy with the Father, because in knowing Him with ongoing experience, we discover who we are.

And because our true identity is eternally tied to the One who called us each by name, *in Him* we have access to discern the value system of the kingdom, which calibrates our default approach to everyday life and provides strategies and hope for the challenges that come our way. It anchors our hearts in a superior reality where His goodness and mercy follow us each day; where with Him, nothing is impossible; where solutions are provided before problems are encountered. And because of Him, even what appears to be hopeless and lost finds not only redemption but also restoration.

Practically speaking, therefore, if receiving our true identity comes by way of abiding, how does this play out day to day? Fundamentally, it requires regular time alone with the Lord, in the Scriptures, and in our community of believers where formation of our spirits and souls takes place. And as we abide in Him, we mature and bear fruit. In many ways, I believe this is the greatest call to believers: to grow in maturity because of the inheritance and call to sonship our loving Father has given to us.[10]

Everything we have discussed in this book—from breaking free from the cycle of pain and unhinging our souls from shame, to learning the art of surrender, to traversing the pathway to peace, to grieving and renewing our minds—takes place as we abide on the Vine because of who we are in Him and because of Christ in us, the hope of glory![11] And most assuredly, it happens as we take courage, get up, and answer His call to be transformed from the inside out. Knowing who we are in Christ is therefore the hinge to all other facets of this journey toward wholeness.

THE TRAP OF SELF-CREATION

There is a caveat to this message of identity, however: Our true identity will never result from self-creation. You see, contrary to the cultural narrative of the day, we will never find the truth of who we are through introspection or self-actualization; we will find it only as we abide in Christ, branch to Vine. *Jesus* is the Author and Finisher of our faith.[12] And as my friend Jamie Winship says, "When we take our eyes off Jesus, . . . we stop abiding and we become separate from truth. This separation results in a descent into falsehood. This descent, unchecked, whether gradual or rapid, is inevitable and often destructive."[13]

And in no subtle fashion, falsehood and destruction are on display—and *marketed*—in the secular humanistic agenda presently playing out in culture. The exaltation of self-creation has forged a path to hijack the foundation of God-designed identity in humanity. According to the prescription of postmodern ethics in our culture of moral relativism, the locus of one's authority is the "self," and the framework for *right* and *wrong* is relative to an individual's perception and lived experiences. "As long as no one gets hurt, you do you" is the rationale. That methodology not only is problematic, of course, but also includes an agenda that is as overt as it is lethal.

Let's take this a step further to understand the implications of this cultural moment. When we forsake the ways of our Creator/ Designer, we forget our design (our identity). And when we forget our design, we abdicate our purpose. When we abdicate our purpose, we ignore our innate function and thus forsake the responsibility for which we all will someday give an account before the Lord.[14] Sadly, it's no wonder we've found ourselves trapped in a collective state of neurosis at a level we've not seen before. For all the messaging about "living your truth" and "following your heart," are people getting healthier? Freer? Experiencing more wholeness? No. The rate of anxiety and depression in this generation has not waned. But we should not be taken by surprise in this matter either.

Isaiah prophesied, "Behold, darkness shall cover the earth, and thick darkness the peoples; but the LORD will arise upon you, and his glory will be seen upon you."[15] This is why identity matters— knowing who *we* are because of who *He* is. It isn't simply so that we can live "the good life," whatever that means in our current cultural context. It's so that we will live an abundant, fruitful life of faithfulness to the One who called us each by name to provide solutions for our orphaned, broken, hurting society, desperate for union with the Father. Thus, as we've said repeatedly, our most potent work will begin as we abide on the Vine.

We need to reference this cultural rubric in the context of

transformation because of how many of us respond when we are deep in pain or endeavoring to navigate our way through life after trauma. As we've explored, the wisdom of this age tells us to look inward, not upward. But when we reach for identity, truth, and clarity within ourselves, it's like pulling water from a broken cistern.[16] Yet we will find the transformation we truly desire only as we seek the face *and the ways* of the One who created us.

> The wisdom of this age tells us to look inward, not upward. But when we reach for identity, truth, and clarity within ourselves, it's like pulling water from a broken cistern.

We will know ourselves when we know Him. The psalmist gave us language for this reorientation of the soul when he wrote, "I lift up my eyes to the hills. From where does my help come? My help comes from the LORD, who made heaven and earth. He will not let your foot be moved; he who keeps you will not slumber."[17] Translation: Not a moment of your life is outside His watchful care, even when you don't feel it. We can draw great assurance from this.

Remember that our thoughts and feelings don't necessarily validate truth; they validate our *perceptions* of truth. Therefore, in your fervent pursuit of healing and transformation, look upward with the eyes of your heart, not inward. Doing this means we must release both the maniacal drive for control of our lives and the timing and process of our transformation after loss or disappointment. You can't fix yourself by yourself, nor can you find your true self within yourself. In fact, if you want to find your life, you have to let go.

SELF-DENIAL IS THE COST

Jesus told his disciples, "If anyone would come after me, let him deny himself and take up his cross and follow me. For whoever would save his life will lose it, but whoever loses his life for my sake will find it."[18] In an age obsessed with self-creation, self-denial is sacrilege. So, after having unpacked what it means to receive (not conceive) our true identity, are we now confronted with a contradiction of principle? Not at all.

Self-denial isn't about abandoning the true identity ascribed to you by your Creator in your mother's womb or the God-given purpose for which you were created to bring Him glory and extend His kingdom. Remember that it was Paul who wrote, "We are his workmanship, created in Christ Jesus for good works, which God prepared beforehand, that we should walk in them."[19] So, what *is* Jesus talking about?

Self-denial is about taking yourself out of the center of the narrative and allowing the Author and Finisher of your faith to occupy that place of leadership *and lordship* in your life. It involves purging your soul of the attachments that serve as substitutes for His presence and counterfeit agents of effective formation. Essentially, these soul attachments distract us and untether us from simple childlike trust in the name of the Lord and undermine our purposes in this life.

So, how do we walk in this reality? We walk in step with the Holy Spirit as our leader by setting our minds and *keeping them set* on truth. Here's Paul again: "If then you have been raised with Christ, seek the things that are above, where Christ is, seated at the right hand of God. Set your minds on things that are above, not on things that are on earth. For you have died, and your life is hidden with Christ in God."[20] This deep work of formation, this denial of self, is a transfer of trust. It is a change of mindset. And it is an exchange of identity in which, by losing sight of ourselves, we will receive true and everlasting life in Christ.

TRANSFORMED TO TRANSFORM

With this personal cost of surrender comes the great privilege of co-laboring with the Lord for the advancement of His kingdom in the rebuilding of nations, systems, and people groups. Having been restored and transformed, we will be used by the Lord to restore and transform others by the power of His Spirit at work in us.

This is the great testimony Isaiah prophesied about in chapter 61, which Jesus proclaimed in Luke 4 as His public ministry assignment. Have a look at the Lord's intentions in Isaiah:

> The Spirit of the Lord GOD is upon me,
>> because the LORD has anointed me
> to bring good news to the poor;
>> he has sent me to bind up the brokenhearted,
> to proclaim liberty to the captives,
>> and the opening of the prison to those who are bound;
> to proclaim the year of the LORD's favor,
>> and the day of vengeance of our God;
> to comfort all who mourn;
> to grant to those who mourn in Zion—
>> to give them a beautiful headdress instead of ashes,
> the oil of gladness instead of mourning,
>> the garment of praise instead of a faint spirit;
> that they may be called oaks of righteousness,
>> the planting of the LORD, that he may be glorified.
> They shall build up the ancient ruins;
>> they shall raise up the former devastations;
> they shall repair the ruined cities,
>> the devastations of many generations.[21]

Those who will rebuild the ancient ruins, raise up the former desolations, and repair the ruined cities are those who were bound up, comforted, set free, and ultimately transformed only a few verses earlier. That is remarkable! And this is our testimony: Having been transformed from the inside out, our lives will bear witness to the eternal truth that He and He alone restores the brokenhearted. He gives us a new name. He rebuilds those that others said were hopeless. He adopts the abandoned and forsaken. And He heals what cannot be erased! So, will you set yourself apart for a generation that is hungry and desperately thirsty for true life?

With our identity secured in Christ comes a clarion call to broker the realities of the kingdom, from heaven to earth, to people who are in need as we go about our everyday lives. But to perceive these needs, we must see Him first. We must look upward, not inward! If this is your desire, position yourself afresh before the Lord and answer the following question with trust and confidence in His power, wisdom, and goodness: *Who do you think you are?*

> He and He alone restores the brokenhearted. He gives us a new name. He rebuilds those that others said were hopeless. He adopts the abandoned and forsaken. And He heals what cannot be erased!

When you and I met on the first few pages of this book, I essentially told you that transformation isn't a destination; it's a door that opens to the ongoing work of the Holy Spirit in our lives until we reach eternity. And by now, I hope you see that principle even more clearly than when our time together began. Transformation and healing what can't be erased involves and affects us, but in the view of God's eternal purposes, it isn't fully about us. We simply aren't the point of our own stories. We are transformed . . . *to transform.* We are restored . . . *to restore.* And we are rebuilt from the inside out . . . *to rebuild* for the glory of the Lord in our generation.

At the time of this writing, it was ten years earlier, almost to the day, that the greatest losses of my life occurred. If you had asked me then if I could see hope for restoration in my future, I would have scoffed. The last ten years have been hard yet bittersweet as I have fought for every word you have read in the twelve chapters of this book. But I sit before you today with a testimony of restoration and of the goodness of the Lord. Let my life be a living example to you that the Lord is absolutely faithful and undeniably trustworthy.

And yet this work is not finished. None of us have to move on from the pain and losses of yesterday. But if we're going to steward this short life of ours, we must move forward. Healing what can never be erased in life is possible. I'm living proof of it.

And now, it's your turn.

PERSONALIZE IT

THE POINT

Receiving our true identity is the fruit of abiding, not striving. We will know ourselves when we know Him, for our real lives are hidden in Christ.

THE PROMPT

Though brokenness may have happened to you somewhere in your past, can you recognize ways in which "broken" became the identity through which you see yourself and your relation to the Lord? What deliberate steps will you take to pursue inner healing for this broken narrative? And as a consequence of experiencing the healing love of your Father, answer this question: Who do you think you are?

THE POSTURE

If you want to receive and walk in your true identity, you must answer the call of the Lord. You must come out of hiding. You must take courage and get up by faith to receive what He has prepared for you: restoration, hope, and healing from the sting of death and loss from the seasons that cannot be erased from your life's story.

THE PRAYER

Lord, I want to walk uprightly in my true identity. Teach my heart to fix my focus on You when I am baited to substitute the joy of abiding in Your presence with self-centeredness, insecurity, a victim mentality, pride, or self-promotion. I willingly take myself out of the center of the narrative and give You Your rightful place as my leader and my Lord. I give You every area of my life that represents lameness. Restore me to wholeness. I come fearlessly, boldly, and confidently to the King's table to receive the identity You gave me when You knit me together in my mother's womb. What a great privilege it is. I thank You for this invitation, and I will steward it well for Your glory. Amen.

CONCLUSION

It's a Saturday evening in late October as I write these final words. But what I could never have planned for is that today is exactly eight years, nearly to the *hour,* from when the Lord responded to my prayer by asking, "What do you want Me to do for you?" As you know, His question was not one of curiosity or ignorance to my need; rather, it was rhetorical. Was I willing to take responsibility for my life by no longer finding sufficiency in my deficiencies? And though my answer was yes, I didn't know where to start. But He did. "Take courage and get up," He replied, "because I'm calling you." And that He did—to a journey of transformation by the power of His Spirit that produced not only the change I desired but also a testimony of His goodness and faithfulness to heal what could not be erased from my life experiences in my own strength.

> Take courage.
> Get up. He is
> calling you.

    Take courage. Get up. He is calling you. Those eight words never fail to resonate within me. In many ways, I believe they embody the dynamic work of transformation in our spirits, souls, and bodies, let alone thread together the thesis of this entire book. And because transformation is a daily process that will last a lifetime, not an in-a-day experience, we must take courage, get up from everything that is holding us down, and heed His calling to steward our lives for the sake of His purposes each day. Therefore, the most tragic ending to our time together would be for you to walk away from this book and appreciate it as good information alone. Lasting change requires consistent action.

Take courage. Get up. He's calling you.

Taking courage requires a strong spirit. It is courage not of our own making but rather birthed in trust and confidence in the Lord's power, wisdom, and goodness. We don't often perceive our need for courage on the mountaintops of life when we're experiencing victory. We need courage when adversity and loss challenge the steadfast faithfulness of the Lord.

Getting up requires ability. Those whose spirits are strong, whose emblematic banners are raised to declare that they are "more than conquerors," get up from the woundedness of the past. Their scars tell stories of God's faithfulness to redeem and restore what others said was unredeemable and impossible to turn around. And when we get up *from*, we clothe ourselves in robes of righteousness, in garments of praise, so that we will get up *for* our purposes in Him.

Heeding His call requires our firm yes. It's an act of both desire and intention. And that's just it: We don't have to say yes. We don't *have* to take courage or get up after disappointment and loss. But what's at stake is the healing of what can't be erased from our stories.

No longer should you live satisfied with defeat. Brokenness may have happened, but "broken" is not who you are. Now the invitation is at hand: to be transformed and restored from the inside out, in your spirit, soul, and body, even after the most unimaginable pain. Why? So that you will be one who stands up to declare with confidence that He who began a good work in you will be faithful to bring it to completion. To declare that He is your redeemer and restorer, father, healer. That He is eternally good. That having been transformed, you will follow His call to partner with Him for the transformation of your generation. Those who ran before us carried this mandate—men and women like Joseph, Esther, and Daniel. Thus, I pray for you Paul's words:

> May the God of peace himself sanctify you completely, and may your whole spirit and soul and body be kept blameless at the coming of our Lord Jesus Christ. He who calls you is faithful; he will surely do it.[1]

Faithful is He who calls you to Himself. He will do it. He will heal what can't be erased. So today, take courage and get up. He's calling you.

I believe in you.

A QUICK-START GUIDE TO RENEWING THE MIND
(THE SEED METHOD)

As stated in chapter 11, the goal of this exercise, the SEED Method, is to secure our thoughts, examine their origin, expose them to truth, and decide how to respond in accordance with truth. In doing so, we position ourselves for transformation by the renewal of our minds, just as Paul wrote in Romans 12:2. You can use this page as a template for your work:

Secure a dominant anxious thought in the forefront of your mind so that you can maintain conscious awareness of it.

_____

_____

_____

_____

_____

_____

Examine the motivating factors of that specific thought with the leading of the Holy Spirit. This is an effort to trace the breadcrumbs of the anxious thought and discover and diagnose the root of any believed lie that is keeping the underlying fear response alive.

_____

_____

_____

_____

_____

Expose that thought (and the attached lie) to truth, which will uproot its influence from your mind. How is this accomplished? With Scripture.

_____

_____

_____

_____

Decide to consistently place your focus on the truth of the Word, which will begin the process of installing a new thought into your mind. The Word of God, by the Holy Spirit, contains the power to change your life from the inside out.

_____

_____

_____

_____

_____

ACKNOWLEDGMENTS

———————

Behind this book is a group of selfless, generous, intelligent, creative, committed, caring, and incredibly talented people who have both championed and challenged me along the way. Since there's no way I could have done this without their guidance and expertise, I'd like to thank them by name.

To my literary agent, Trinity McFadden, and to the entire team at The Bindery Agency (most especially Alex Field and Ingrid Beck), thank you for believing in me and investing in me. Trinity, you're a gift to my life. After our very first meeting, I knew that I knew (that I knew) I wanted to write books with you in my corner. Your industry acumen, spirit of excellence, tenacity, intuition, and commitment to this project have blown me away. I couldn't have done this without you, nor would I have wanted to. Thank you, my friend. Let's do it again soon.

To the incredible people at WaterBrook and Penguin Random House, thank you for this opportunity. It is quite literally a dream come true. To my editor, Susan Tjaden, you've made me a better writer. Your wisdom and keen understanding of what makes a book commercially relevant has changed my life. No one has made me think about a sentence or a turn to the reader quite like you. I'm excited for what's ahead! To my copy editors, Tracey Moore and Helen Macdonald, your trophies are on the way. Your professionalism, commitment to literary excellence, and theological sharpness have been a gift to me and to this writing process. Laura Barker, thank you for your belief in this book and for every nudge toward precision and effectiveness. And to the New York team at Penguin Random House, most certainly Tina Constable, thank you!

To Dr. John Delony, thank you for writing the foreword to this book. Your words are as generous and kind as you are. Your friendship is an anchor in my life. I believe in you. You're helping people emerge out of the ashes of their own lives. I'm thrilled to watch it happen and am cheering you on. Love you, brother.

To Dave and Ann Wilson and Cody and Jenna Wilson, the four of you have made an indelible mark on my life in the last nine years. Running with you has been one of the greatest privileges of my journey thus far. I love you all.

To Dave and Connie, goodness. There's no telling where I would be without you. Your leadership, belief, challenge, and counsel have been a constant catalyst for transformation in my life. Wednesday is my favorite day of the week because of you two. I'm forever grateful.

To Pastor Loren, for over thirty years, I've had the privilege of sitting under your leadership. It's an honor to be called one of your spiritual sons. In many ways, this book—*and the fruit of my life*—is a by-product of your ministry. I believe thirty years' worth of seeds fell on good ground. I pray that I continue to steward my life with the steadfastness, integrity, quiet confidence in the Lord, commitment to the Scriptures, and tenderness of heart that you have so brilliantly modeled. I love you. Thank you.

To the men and women who've encouraged me, empowered me, and sharpened me in my work within the last few years: Carey Nieuwhof, John Eldredge, John and Lisa Bevere, Addison Bevere, Jordan Raynor, Caleb Kaltenbach, Jamie and Donna Winship, Lee

Cummings, Michele Cushatt, Hannah Brencher, Dr. Curt Thompson, Debra Fileta, Dr. John Townsend, Gary Thomas, Nona Jones, Levi Lusko, David Nurse, Dr. Dharius Daniels, Jason Wilson, Shanon Stowe, Robin Barnett, and so many more, thank you.

To my family and friends, you've watched this story unfold up close. Your commitment to me, even in the valley, continues to bless me. I'm so thankful for you and love you all.

To my listeners, say it with me: "Transformation beats self-help . . . all day long." It's a joy to serve you each and every week.

To Dad, while this book highlights a specific season in my life where pain and loss abounded, in no way does it minimize the sacrifice, love, provision, and example you gave to me throughout my entire upbringing. And that's why I want to acknowledge you here. Your commitment to do what is right because it is the right thing to do has always inspired me in the same way. Between mopping floors at our school after your already taxing day job to refereeing high school basketball games to turning down a promotion just for more time with Carmen and me, your "whatever it takes" work ethic provided a shining example for me to follow. I'm so thankful, and I love you so much.

And to Pops and Carmen. You know this story better than anyone else because you lived it with me. Thank you for fiercely championing my life, for sacrificing for me, for loving me when I was at rock bottom, and for staying by my side without wavering, especially in the last decade. Here we are, nearly thirty years since it all began, and though we all have scars, we have seen the faithfulness of the Lord in our lives. He is undeniably our restorer. Mom is so proud; I'm sure of it. I love you with my whole heart.

NOTES

Start Here

1. "Anxiety Disorders—Facts and Statistics," Anxiety & Depression Association of America, updated October 28, 2022, https://adaa.org/understanding-anxiety/facts-statistics#Facts%20and%20Statistics; "Anxiety Disorders," National Alliance on Mental Illness, reviewed December 2017, www.nami.org/About-Mental-Illness/Mental-Health-Conditions/Anxiety-Disorders.

2. Giancarlo Pasquini and Scott Keeter, "At Least Four-in-Ten U.S. Adults Have Faced High Levels of Psychological Distress During COVID-19 Pandemic," Pew Research Center, December 12, 2022, www.pewresearch.org/fact-tank/2022/12/12/at-least-four-in-ten-u-s-adults-have-faced-high-levels-of-psychological-distress-during-covid-19-pandemic.

3. Pasquini and Keeter, "At Least Four-in-Ten."

4. "Post-Traumatic Stress Disorder (PTSD) 2022," National Institutes of Health, https://hr.nih.gov/working-nih/civil/post-traumatic-stress-disorder-ptsd-2022.

5. Isaiah 60:2.

6. *Strong's Exhaustive Concordance,* s.v. "2822. *choshek,*" Bible Hub, https://biblehub.com/hebrew/2822.htm.

7. J. Alec Motyer, *The Prophecy of Isaiah: An Introduction and Commentary* (Downers Grove, Ill.: InterVarsity, 1993), 494.

8. Motyer, *Prophecy of Isaiah,* 494.

9. Isaiah 60:1, AMPC.

CHAPTER 1:
"HOLE"-NESS

1. Adam J. Waxman et al., "Racial Disparities in Incidence and Outcome in Multiple Myeloma: A Population Based Study," *Blood* 116, no. 25 (September 2010): 5501–6. www.ncbi.nlm.nih.gov/pmc/articles/PMC3031400.

2. Abdul Wali Khan et al., "Far and Few Between: Early Onset Multiple Myeloma in 26-Year-Old Female," *Cureus* 12, no. 8 (August 2020): 9588, www.ncbi.nlm.nih.gov/pmc/articles/PMC7478686.

CHAPTER 2:
YOU ARE NOT ENOUGH

1. Though the mechanics of exerting willpower (set your intention, create a plan, and then put the plan into action) are widely known, I want to credit Alexander Loyd as being one of the first to articulate this "blueprint": Alexander Loyd, *Beyond Willpower: The Secret Principle to Achieving Success in Life, Love, and Happiness* (New York: Harmony Books, 2015), 3, 28.

2. Loyd, *Beyond Willpower,* 5.

3. Loyd, *Beyond Willpower,* 5.

4. "Stress Effects on the Body," American Psychological Association, last modified March 8, 2023, www.apa.org/topics/stress/body.

5. Bruce S. McEwen, "Neurobiological and Systemic Effects of Chronic Stress," *Chronic Stress (Thousand Oaks),* no. 1 (January–December 2017), www.ncbi.nlm.nih.gov/pmc/articles/PMC5573220.

6. McEwen, "Neurobiological and Systemic Effects."

7. McEwen, "Neurobiological and Systemic Effects."

8. "Understanding the Stress Response," Harvard Health Publishing, July 6, 2020, www.health.harvard.edu/staying-healthy/understanding-the-stress-response.

9. Loyd, *Beyond Willpower*, 29.

10. "Protect Your Brain from Stress," Harvard Health Publishing, February 15, 2021, www.health.harvard.edu/mind-and-mood/protect-your -brain-from-stress.

11. "Protect Your Brain."

12. "Protect Your Brain."

13. Bruce H. Lipton, *The Biology of Belief: Unleashing the Power of Consciousness, Matter, and Miracles* (Carlsbad, Calif.: Hay House, 2008), 176.

14. Lipton, *The Biology of Belief*, 229.

15. Considering what Paul wrote in Romans 6:1–11 about the new nature we share because of the atoning, finished work of Jesus Christ, many scholars contend that in chapter 7, he was speaking about his wrestle between reason and passion not in the present tense but in diatribe style, vividly describing his *past* life under the law. Supporting this theory, Craig Keener asserted, "A number of scholars today also argue that this passage is *prosopopoiia*, in which one rhetorically speaks with the voice of another character, 'impersonating' a person or a thing, in this case Adamic humanity or (perhaps more likely) Israel under the law." *The IVP Bible Background Commentary: New Testament*, 2nd ed. (Downers Grove, Ill.: IVP Academic, 2014), 437. And thus, we can consider a broader narrative in this context: The power to live rightly is purely a gift of God's grace, not a feat of our own effort. In his commentary on Romans 7:15, Keener explained that "philosophers spoke of an internal conflict between the reason and the passions; Jewish teachers spoke of a conflict between the good and evil impulse. Either could identify with Paul's contrast between his mind or reason—knowing what was right—and his members in which passions or the evil impulse worked. The language of moral helplessness here resembles some tragic depictions of passion overpowering reason." *IVP Bible Background Commentary*, 438.

16. Proverbs 4:23, NIV.

17. *Strong's Concordance*, s.v. "3820. *leb*," Bible Hub, https://biblehub .com/hebrew/3820.htm.

18. Keener, *IVP Bible Background Commentary*, 293.

19. Proverbs 27:17.

20. Matthew 6:21.

21. Paul's use of the word *sons* was not intended to exclude women.

22. James 4:14.

23. James 1:5.

CHAPTER 3:
THE BROKEN SPIRIT

1. Genesis 12:1–2.

2. Exodus 14:13.

3. Exodus 1:11–14.

4. Numbers 13:27–28.

5. Numbers 13:30.

6. Numbers 13:32–33.

7. Numbers 14:2–4.

8. Numbers 14:7–9.

9. Numbers 14:11–12.

10. Exodus 33:11.

11. Numbers 14:15–19.

12. Numbers 14:22–23.

13. Numbers 14:24.

14. The Bible, on numerous occasions throughout the Old and New Testaments, teaches that we are triune beings, composed of spirit, soul, and body. Interestingly, some scholars argue that we are not three-part but two-part beings: a composite of spirit-soul (the immaterial) and the body (the material).

   My angle in this context isn't to contemplate the delineation among our parts or explore the nuances of the ancient language from which words such as *spirit* and *soul* were derived. Hebrews 4:12 says, "The Word that God speaks is alive and full of power [making it active, operative, energizing, and effective]; it is sharper than any two-edged sword, penetrating to the dividing line of the breath of life (soul) and [the immortal] spirit, and of joints and marrow [of the deepest parts of our nature], exposing and sifting and analyzing and judging the very thoughts and purposes of the heart" (AMPC). Therefore, I believe the interconnectedness of soul and spirit is such that only the living Word of God (the *logos*) can separate the two. Instead, I'm focusing on the fact that the immaterial part of us is essential and complex. It affects every other area of our lives and, when wounded, can collapse our physical and emotional health and compromise our potential in life. That said, we will work from the framework that we are each one whole person, comprised of three distinct yet interconnected parts: spirit, soul, and body.

15. *Strong's Concordance*, s.v. "7307. *ruach*," Bible Hub, https://biblehub .com/hebrew/7307.htm.

16. Exodus 1:11, 13–14.

17. Laura van Dernoot Lipsky, stated in Ed Yong, "What Happens When Americans Can Finally Exhale: The Pandemic's Mental Wounds Are Still Wide Open," *The Atlantic*, May 20, 2021, www.theatlantic.com/ health/archive/2021/05/pandemic-trauma-summer/618934.

18. Hebrews 3:10–11.

19. John 15:1–7.

20. Romans 8:35–39.

21. Ronald Rolheiser, *The Shattered Lantern: Rediscovering a Felt Presence of God* (New York: Crossroad, 2004), 22.

22. Proverbs 11:14.

23. Job 17:1.

24. *Strong's Concordance*, s.v. "2254. *chabal*," Bible Hub, https://biblehub .com/hebrew/2254.htm.

25. Søren Kierkegaard, *The Sickness unto Death: A Christian Psychological Exposition for Upbuilding and Awakening*, ed. and trans. Howard V. Hong and Edna H. Hong (Princeton, N.J.: Princeton University Press, 1980).

26. Psalm 139:14.

27. Genesis 3:12.

28. Exodus 14:11–12.

29. Bessel A. van der Kolk, *The Body Keeps the Score: Brain, Mind, and Body in the Healing of Trauma* (New York: Penguin, 2014), 53.

30. Van der Kolk, *The Body Keeps the Score,* 53.

31. 3 John 2.

32. Joel 2:25, AMPC.

33. Proverbs 4:23, AMPC.

34. Timothy Keller, "The Wounded Spirit," sermon, Redeemer Presbyterian Church, December 5, 2004, New York, YouTube video, 9:21, www.youtube.com/watch?v=pkL3R27ZV1o&t=22s.

35. Keller, "The Wounded Spirit," 9:30.

CHAPTER 4:
WHEN SHAME ARRIVES

1. Curt Thompson, *The Soul of Shame: Retelling the Stories We Believe About Ourselves* (Downers Grove, Ill.: IVP Books, 2015), 21.

2. Thompson, *The Soul of Shame,* 22.

3. Brené Brown, *Atlas of the Heart: Mapping Meaningful Connection and the Language of Human Experience* (New York: Random House, 2021), 137.

4. Brené Brown provides a similar list in *Atlas of the Heart* (pages 136–37). Thus, I want to credit her for inspiring my own examples.

5. In chapter 6, you'll be introduced to a man named Dave and his wife, Connie, who have been instrumental in my journey to healing and wholeness. The description of shame as believing that we are "uniquely and fatally flawed" is Dave's.

6. Genesis 2:25.

7. Christopher Cook, "The Soul of Shame and What Shame Does to You (feat. Curt Thompson, MD)," December 2, 2020, *Win Today with Christopher Cook,* podcast, 14:44, 16:04, https://wintoday.tv/episode221.

8. Although Scripture specifies that Adam was with Eve during her discourse with the serpent (see Genesis 3:6), it's also clear in the text that the inquisition initiated by the serpent was directed at Eve (see Genesis 3:1). In so doing, the serpent essentially isolated her in conversation from Adam. First Timothy 2:14 validates the

consequence of this isolation: "Adam was not deceived, but the woman was deceived and became a transgressor." Was Adam innocent in this whole situation? Absolutely not. But in our context, Eve is our point of reference when illustrating the strength of isolation and deception regarding the inception and exacerbation of shame. Another example of isolation in the garden is found in Genesis 3:8. Following their disobedient act, Adam and Eve sewed fig leaves together to cover their nakedness (3:7). And in verse eight, Scripture says, "They heard the sound of the Lord God walking in the garden in the cool of the day, and the man and his wife hid themselves from the presence of the Lord God among the trees of the garden." The point is that shame causes us to hide, and when we hide (isolate/separate), shame thrives. Thus, two avenues by which shame establishes a footing in our lives are isolation (separateness) and deception.

9. 2 Corinthians 10:5, AMPC.

10. James 1:13–15.

11. Genesis 3:2–3.

12. Genesis 3:4–5.

13. Genesis 3:7.

14. Thompson, *The Soul of Shame,* 22 (emphasis mine).

15. Romans 8:37.

16. Psalm 139:23.

17. Psalm 139:13.

18. Matthew 11:28, AMPC.

CHAPTER 5:
HOW SHAME THRIVES

1. Since I first learned about these manifestations of shame from my friend and mentor Jamie Winship, I want to credit him for the intelligence.

2. Brené Brown, *Atlas of the Heart: Mapping Meaningful Connection and the Language of Human Experience* (New York: Random House, 2021), 137.

3. "The fingerprints of the Enemy are secrecy and shame" is a phrase used by Jamie Winship.

4. Genesis 3:12.

5. Genesis 3:13.

6. Psalm 104:2.

7. "Does Genesis 3 Suggest That Adam and Eve's Fig-leaf Loincloths (v. 7) Were Unable to Cover Nakedness, Unlike the Tunics of Skin (v. 21)?," Biblical Hermeneutics, Stack Exchange, August 2021, https://hermeneutics.stackexchange.com/questions/66983/does-genesis-3-suggest-that-adam-and-eves-fig-leaf-loincloths-v-7-were-unabl.

8. Genesis 1:28.

9. Romans 8:37.

10. Romans 14:12.

11. Genesis 3:1.

12. Curt Thompson, *The Soul of Shame: Retelling the Stories We Believe About Ourselves* (Downers Grove, Ill.: IVP Books, 2015), 47.

13. 1 John 4:18.

14. Lauri Nummenmaa et al., "Bodily Maps of Emotions," *Proceedings of the National Academy of Sciences of the United States of America* 111, no. 2 (December 30, 2013): 646–51, www.pnas.org/doi/10.1073/pnas.1321664111 (emphasis mine).

15. Olga Khazan, "Mapping How Emotions Manifest in the Body," *The Atlantic,* December 30, 2013, www.theatlantic.com/health/archive/2013/12/mapping-how-emotions-manifest-in-the-body/282713.

16. Nummenmaa et al., "Bodily Maps of Emotions."

17. Heidi L. Dempsey, "A Comparison of the Social-Adaptive Perspective and Functionalist Perspective on Guilt and Shame," *Behavioral Sciences (Basel)* 7, no. 4 (December 11, 2017): 83, www.ncbi.nlm.nih.gov/pmc/articles/PMC5746692.

18. Ashley Abramson, "The Science of Shame," Medium.com, July 22, 2020, https://elemental.medium.com/the-science-of-shame-e1cb32f6f2a.

19. "Protect Your Brain from Stress," Harvard Health Publishing, February 15, 2021, www.health.harvard.edu/mind-and-mood/protect-your-brain-from-stress.

20. Dempsey, "Comparison of the Social-Adaptive Perspective" (emphasis mine).

21. Romans 8:14–17. The term *sonship,* which is not gender specific, refers to our position in relation to the Lord as His adopted children, both male and female. It speaks of our familial identity and our inheritance in the Lord as "fellow heirs with Christ" (Romans 8:17). Just as we all are the bride of Christ, we all are called to sonship.

22. Brown, *Atlas of the Heart,* 137.

23. Brown, *Atlas of the Heart,* 139.

24. Brown, *Atlas of the Heart,* 139.

25. Thompson, *The Soul of Shame,* 121.

26. Thompson, *The Soul of Shame,* 120.

27. Genesis 2:25.

28. David G. Benner, *Surrender to Love: Discovering the Heart of Christian Spirituality* (Downers Grove, Ill.: InterVarsity, 2003), 77.

29. Psalm 24:3–4.

30. Benner, *Surrender to Love,* 77–78.

31. Isaiah 61:3.

32. Isaiah 61:7.

CHAPTER 6:
THE ART OF SURRENDER

1. Jamie Winship shared this exact statement with me in a personal conversation and also on episode 298 of my podcast: "Jamie Winship on How to Live Fearless in Your True Identity," June 15, 2022, *Win Today with Christopher Cook,* podcast, https://wintoday.tv/episode298.

2. I've heard many counselors and speakers, such as Henry Cloud, Christine Caine, and my own therapist, share derivatives of this statement, so I cannot pinpoint an exact source. And even the statement in this book is a derivative of a derivative.

3. Mark 10:50, AMPC.

4. Mark 10:51–52, AMPC.

5. Jamie Winship, *Living Fearless: Exchanging the Lies of the World for the Liberating Truth of God* (Grand Rapids, Mich.: Revell, 2022), 47.

6. Winship, *Living Fearless,* 47.

7. *Thayer's Greek Lexicon,* s.v. "3670. *homologeó,*" Bible Hub, https://biblehub.com/greek/3670.htm.

8. Proverbs 4:23, NIV.

9. See 2 Samuel 12 for the details of the confrontation.

10. Jeremiah 1:7–8.

11. Winship, *Living Fearless,* 47–48.

12. James 5:16–18.

13. Romans 8:37.

14. Isaiah 61:3.

15. Psalm 51:17.

16. Psalm 139:7.

17. Psalm 139:12.

18. Psalm 56:8.

19. Hosea 10:12.

20. 2 Timothy 2:21.

21. Psalm 16:11.

22. John 15:4–7.

23. Sherri Seligson, "A Scientific Look at the Branches, Vine, and Grafting in the Bible," March 3, 2015, www.sherriseligson.com/blog/a-scientific-look-at-the-branches-vine-and-grafting-in-the-bible.

24. Isaiah 53:5.

25. John 2:7–8.

26. Matthew 11:28–30.

27. Hebrews 13:8.

28. Hebrews 13:5.

29. 1 Thessalonians 5:23–24.

NOTES239

CHAPTER 7:
NECESSARY GRIEVING

1. Colin Murray Parkes, *Bereavement: Studies of Grief in Adult Life,* 3rd ed. (New York: Routledge, 1996), 6.

2. D. A. Carson, *How Long, O Lord? Reflections on Suffering and Evil,* 2nd ed. (Grand Rapids, Mich.: Baker Academic, 2006), 67.

3. David Kessler, *Finding Meaning: The Sixth Stage of Grief* (New York: Scribner, 2019), 29.

4. Kessler, *Finding Meaning,* 29.

5. Isaiah 53:3.

6. Psalm 147:3.

7. John H. Walton, Victor H. Matthews, and Mark W. Chavalas, *The IVP Bible Background Commentary: Old Testament* (Downers Grove, Ill.: InterVarsity, 2000), 281.

8. 1 Samuel 1:8.

9. 1 Samuel 1:15.

10. Hebrews 12:15.

11. 1 Samuel 1:16.

12. "The Nature and Purpose of Grief," Highlands Funeral Home, www.highlandsfuneralhome.com/the-nature-and-purpose-of-grief.

13. Job 1:1.

14. Job 1:21, NLT.

15. Job 2:7.

16. Job 2:9.

17. Job 2:10.

18. 1 Thessalonians 4:13.

19. Curt Thompson, *The Soul of Desire: Discovering the Neuroscience of Longing, Beauty, and Community* (Downers Grove, Ill.: InterVarsity, 2021), 73.

20. Kessler, *Finding Meaning,* 1.

21. Kessler, *Finding Meaning*, 1.

22. Kessler, *Finding Meaning*, 2.

23. Kessler, *Finding Meaning*, 2.

24. Hebrews 13:5.

25. Kessler, *Finding Meaning*, 3.

26. Kate Placzek, "Understanding a Broken Heart—The Physiology of Grief," The ZRT Laboratory Blog, August 28, 2020, www.zrtlab.com/blog/archive/the-physiology-of-grief.

27. Placzek, "Understanding a Broken Heart."

28. Proverbs 4:23, NLT.

29. Isaiah 61:3.

30. Romans 8:28.

31. Brené Brown, *Atlas of the Heart: Mapping Meaningful Connection and the Language of Human Experience* (New York: Random House, 2021), 91.

32. "Complicated Grief," Ricky, Inc., https://rickyinc.org/grief. This link provides the information previously found on Columbia University's website The Center for Prolonged Grief. Unfortunately, just prior to the publication of this book, Columbia removed the original link (along with the definition for "complicated grief"), so I am referring to this secondary source.

33. Kessler, *Finding Meaning*, 10.

34. Kessler, *Finding Meaning*, 10.

35. Kessler, *Finding Meaning*, 2.

36. Bill Johnson, "The Healing Power of Grief," *Charisma*, January 5, 2023, https://charismamag.com/jan-feb-2023/the-healing-power-of-grief.

CHAPTER 8:
THE PATHWAY TO PEACE

1. John Lennon, "Imagine," *Imagine*, Apple Records, 1971, www.songfacts.com/lyrics/john-lennon/imagine.

2. John 14:27.

3. J. Alec Motyer, *The Prophecy of Isaiah: An Introduction & Commentary* (Downers Grove, Ill.: IVP Academic, 1993), 214.

4. "Peace-Shalom (Hebrew Word Study)," Precept Austin, December 17, 2022, www.preceptaustin.org/shalom_-_definition.

5. "Peace-Eirene (Greek Word Study)," Precept Austin, August 20, 2016, www.preceptaustin.org/peace_eirene.

6. Craig S. Keener, *The Gospel of John: A Commentary,* vol. 2 (Peabody, Mass.: Hendrickson, 2003), 983.

7. Craig S. Keener, *The IVP Bible Background Commentary: New Testament,* 2nd ed. (Downers Grove, Ill.: IVP Academic, 2014), 620.

8. 2 Timothy 3:5.

9. Keener, *IVP Bible Background Commentary,* 620.

10. Hebrews 13:5.

11. Romans 8:28.

12. Proverbs 3:5, AMPC.

13. James 1:8.

14. Ronald Rolheiser, *The Shattered Lantern: Rediscovering a Felt Presence of God* (New York: Crossroad, 2004), 35.

15. John 15:5.

16. William Barclay, *The Letters to the Philippians, Colossians, and Thessalonians,* rev. ed., The Daily Study Bible Series (Louisville, Ky.: Westminster John Knox Press, 1975), 159.

17. 1 Corinthians 3:3–4, NIV.

18. Barclay, *Letters to the Philippians,* 77.

19. An adaptation of John 14:27, AMPC.

20. Philippians 4:6.

21. Barclay, *Letters to the Philippians,* 78.

22. Pastor Bill Johnson from Bethel Church in Redding, California, has made this statement many times throughout the years in various forms. One such reference was found at Bill Johnson, "The Healing Power of Grief," *Charisma,* January 5, 2023, https://charismamag.com/jan-feb-2023/the-healing-power-of-grief.

23. Barclay, *Letters to the Philippians*, 78.

24. Numbers 23:19.

25. Malachi 3:6.

26. Proverbs 3:5–8.

27. Psalm 34:8.

28. Hebrews 13:8.

29. Proverbs 14:12.

30. Rick Warren, *The Purpose-Driven Life* (Grand Rapids, Mich.: Zondervan, 2002), 143.

31. Isaiah 60:1, AMPC.

32. 1 Peter 5:5–10.

33. 1 John 4:18, NKJV.

34. Philippians 4:7.

35. 1 John 3:1, NIV.

36. Psalm 34:10.

37. Psalm 27:13–14.

38. Matthew 6:25–33.

39. Hebrews 4:16, AMPC.

40. Psalm 25:1–2, AMPC.

41. Isaiah 61:7, 10.

42. Psalm 139:17–18.

CHAPTER 9:
CHECK THE GROUND

1. Proverbs 4:23, MSG.

2. *Brown-Driver-Briggs*, s.v. "3820. *leb*," Bible Hub, https://biblehub.com/hebrew/3820.htm.

3. *Strong's Exhaustive Concordance*, s.v. "3820. *leb*," Bible Hub, https://biblehub.com/hebrew/3820.htm.

4. *Thayer's Greek Lexicon*, s.v. "2588. *kardia*," Bible Hub, https://biblehub .com/greek/2588.htm (emphasis mine).

5. Proverbs 23:7, NKJV.

6. Dallas Willard, *Renovation of the Heart: Putting on the Character of Christ* (Colorado Springs: NavPress, 2002), 14.

7. *Strong's Concordance*, s.v. "3308. *merimna*," Bible Hub, https:// biblehub.com/greek/3308.htm.

8. *Thayer's Greek Lexicon*, s.v. "3307. *merizó*," Bible Hub, https:// biblehub.com/greek/3307.htm.

9. Matthew 6:22.

10. James 1:22, AMPC.

11. Proverbs 4:23, NLT.

CHAPTER 10:
WORK THE GROUND

1. Elizabeth A. Stanley, *Widen the Window: Training Your Brain and Body to Thrive During Stress and Recover from Trauma* (New York: Avery, 2019), 14.

2. Stanley, *Widen the Window*, 14.

3. Bessel A. van der Kolk, *The Body Keeps the Score: Brain, Mind, and Body in the Healing of Trauma* (New York: Penguin, 2014), 67 (emphasis mine).

4. 1 Corinthians 3:7–9.

5. John 16:13.

6. Psalm 139:1–10, 13–17.

7. Psalm 139:23–24.

8. Hebrews 12:1, NKJV.

9. Craig S. Keener, *The IVP Bible Background Commentary: New Testament*, 2nd ed. (Downers Grove, Ill.: IVP Academic, 2014), 55.

10. Stanley, *Widen the Window*, 13 (emphasis mine). Please note that the word *mindfulness* in this context is used to simply (and only) describe our need to pay attention and maintain awareness of our thoughts

and emotions in real time. (For more on this subject, please refer to Dr. Henry Cloud's helpful article "Using Mindfulness to Combat Anxiety" at www.boundaries.me/blog/using-mindfulness-to-combat -anxiety.) By no means am I insinuating a connection to (or endorsing) the popular "mindfulness meditation," which has roots in Buddhism and is also connected to New Age practices. I vehemently reject both.

11. Proverbs 27:6.

12. Jill Suttie, "What You Think About Your Emotions Matters," *Greater Good Magazine,* January 8, 2019, https://greatergood.berkeley.edu/ article/item/what_you_think_about_your_emotions_matters.

13. Dallas Willard, *Renovation of the Heart: Putting on the Character of Christ* (Colorado Springs: NavPress, 2002), 33.

14. Romans 12:1–2.

15. Dr. Gloria Willcox, "The Feeling Wheel," *The Gottman Institute,* https://cdn.gottman.com/wp-content/uploads/2020/12/The-Gottman -Institute_The-Feeling-Wheel_v2.pdf.

16. I learned this technique from my friends and mentors Jamie and Donna Winship. I want to credit them for teaching me this valuable practice and methodology, which I am thankful to share in this book.

17. 2 Corinthians 10:5.

18. Alexander Loyd, *The Healing Code: 6 Minutes to Heal the Source of Your Health, Success, or Relationship Issue* (New York: Grand Central, 2010), 14, 97.

19. Van der Kolk, *The Body Keeps the Score,* 45.

20. Psalm 139:13.

21. Psalm 139:23.

22. John 8:32.

CHAPTER 11:
THE POWER OF A TRANSFORMED MIND

1. Psalm 42:11.

2. Ephesians 2:6 says, "He raised us up together with Him and made us sit down together [giving us joint seating with Him] in the heavenly

sphere [by virtue of our being] in Christ Jesus (the Messiah, the Anointed One)" (AMPC). Our perspective about our position in life determines the posture by which we live each day of our lives.

3. Dina Scolan, "Rumination," The OCD and Anxiety Center, March 15, 2021, https://theocdandanxietycenter.com/rumination/ #:~:text=Rumination%20is%20defined%20as%20engaging,to %20solve%20an%20evasive%20problem.

4. Psalm 34:8.

5. Hebrews 13:5.

6. Romans 8:14–16, 29.

7. Jeffrey M. Schwartz and Rebecca Gladding, *You Are Not Your Brain: The Four-Step Solution for Changing Bad Habits, Ending Unhealthy Thinking, and Taking Control of Your Life* (New York: Avery, 2011), 74–75.

8. Caroline Leaf, *Switch On Your Brain: The Key to Peak Happiness, Thinking, and Health* (Grand Rapids, Mich.: Baker, 2013), 19.

9. Proverbs 4:23, NLT.

10. *Brown-Driver-Briggs,* s.v. "3820. *leb,*" Bible Hub, https://biblehub .com/hebrew/3820.htm.

11. Philippians 4:8.

12. I am regularly encouraged by Proverbs 8:17, which says, "I love those who love me, and those who seek me early and diligently shall find me" (AMPC). There is an advantage to filling our minds with truth that calibrates our focus first thing each day.

13. Romans 12:2.

14. Caroline Leaf, *Think, Learn, Succeed: Understanding and Using Your Mind to Thrive at School, the Workplace, and Life* (Grand Rapids, Mich.: Baker, 2018), 38.

15. Leaf, *Switch On Your Brain,* 56.

16. Proverbs 14:30, AMPC.

17. Caroline Leaf, *Who Switched Off My Brain? Controlling Toxic Thoughts and Emotions,* rev. ed. (Southlake, Tex.: Inprov, 2009), 20.

18. Dallas Willard, *Renovation of the Heart: Putting on the Character of Christ* (Colorado Springs: NavPress, 2002), 95.

19. Bessel van der Kolk, *The Body Keeps the Score: Brain, Mind, and Body in the Healing of Trauma* (New York: Penguin, 2014), 177.

20. Willard, *Renovation of the Heart,* 95.

21. The word *hope* is derived from the Greek word *elpis,* which has to do with the expectation of good. For more detail, visit https://biblehub .com/greek/1680.htm.

22. Hebrews 6:19.

23. Contrary to the faulty wisdom of this age, our true identity is not found in and of ourselves but is found hidden in Christ. See Colossians 3:3.

24. Alexander Loyd, *The Healing Code: 6 Minutes to Heal the Source of Your Health, Success, or Relationship Issue* (New York: Grand Central, 2010), 97.

25. 1 Samuel 18:5–7.

26. 1 Samuel 24:1–7; 26:5–12.

27. 1 Samuel 29:5.

28. First Samuel 30:6 says, "David was greatly distressed, for the men spoke of stoning him because the souls of them all were bitterly grieved, each man for his sons and daughters" (AMPC). But David's response was to strengthen and encourage himself in the Lord.

29. Psalm 27:3–5.

30. Caroline Leaf, "The One Mind-Management Technique Required for Sustainable Healing," DrLeaf, December 19, 2021, https://drleaf.com/ blogs/news/the-one-mind-management-technique-required-for -sustainable-healing.

31. Nancy Chick, "Metacognition," Vanderbilt University Center for Teaching, 2013, https://cft.vanderbilt.edu/guides-sub-pages/ metacognition.

32. "Write Your Anxieties Away," Harvard Health Blog, October 13, 2017, www.health.harvard.edu/blog/write-your-anxieties-away -2017101312551.

33. Dr. Caroline Leaf was the first scientist I heard to teach about holding a thought like an object in our hands. Thus, I give her the credit for the illustration.

34. John 16:13; 8:32.

35. Psalm 121:1–2.

36. John 8:44, NIV.

37. 1 John 4:18, AMPC.

38. 2 Corinthians 10:4, AMPC.

39. Romans 8:29, AMPC.

CHAPTER 12:
WHO DO YOU THINK YOU ARE?

1. James F. Masterson, *The Search for the Real Self: Unmasking the Personality Disorders of Our Age* (New York: Free Press, 1988), 67.

2. Brennan Manning, *Abba's Child: The Cry of the Heart for Intimate Belonging* (Colorado Springs: NavPress, 1994), 30.

3. Romans 8:15.

4. Manning, *Abba's Child*, 37–38.

5. David Guzik, "2 Samuel 9—David's Kindness to Mephibosheth," *The Enduring Word Bible Commentary*, https://enduringword.com/bible-commentary/2-samuel-9.

6. 2 Samuel 9:3.

7. Charles Haddon Spurgeon, "May 27th—Morning Reading," *Morning and Evening*, Blue Letter Bible, www.blueletterbible.org/devotionals/me/view.cfm?Date=05/27&body.

8. 2 Samuel 9:8.

9. David G. Benner, *The Gift of Being Yourself: The Sacred Call to Self-Discovery* (Downers Grove, Ill.: InterVarsity, 2015), 83.

10. Romans 8:14–17. Once again, *sonship* is not a gender-specific term; it is indicative of our position in Christ as men and women who have been invited to live as joint heirs with Christ.

11. Colossians 1:27.

12. Hebrews 12:2, NKJV.

13. Jamie Winship, *Living Fearless: Exchanging the Lies of the World for the Liberating Truth of God* (Grand Rapids, Mich.: Revell, 2022), 81.

14. Bill Johnson, "Restored to Design," December 15, 2019, *Bethel Redding Sermon of the Week,* podcast, 3:11, https://podcasts.apple.com/us/podcast/restored-to-design/id1607778827?i=1000549470078.

15. Isaiah 60:2.

16. Jeremiah 2:13.

17. Psalm 121:1–3.

18. Matthew 16:24–25.

19. Ephesians 2:10.

20. Colossians 3:1–3.

21. Isaiah 61:1–4.

CONCLUSION

1. 1 Thessalonians 5:23–24.

ABOUT THE AUTHOR

CHRISTOPHER COOK is a leadership coach, author, and pastor focused on transformation and wholeness. With an aptitude for strategy and execution, his ability to unearth clarity out of complexity drives his mission to help individuals and organizations thrive in their true identity. His work has appeared in various outlets such as *SUCCESS* magazine, and he has spent more than a decade coaching leaders in both the marketplace and nonprofit sectors. His weekly podcast, *Win Today with Christopher Cook*, equips wellness-minded listeners to move beyond the limitations of self-help and instead toward an integrated life of wholeness from the inside out. Pulling from his own experiences of adversity and personal transformation, Christopher's present efforts, embodied by his passion for mental health, emotional health, and spiritual maturity—along with his educational credentials in business administration, leadership, and ministry—have led to helping people experience healing and transformation in their own lives. Connect with Christopher online at wintoday.tv and @wintodaychris on social media.

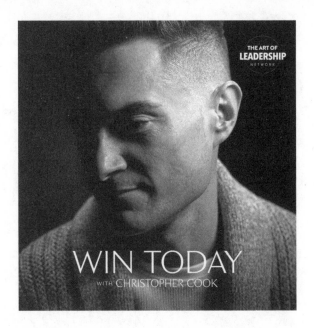

TRANSFORMATION BEATS SELF-HELP

Self-help and life hacks will not turn the key to total life transformation. And creating a plan for transformation is what *Win Today* is all about. Each week, we engage in thought-provoking conversations with world-renowned leaders, bestselling authors, and industry experts who will help you design a roadmap to wholeness in your mental and emotional health and spiritual growth. Subscribe today wherever podcasts are available.

SCAN THE QR CODE TO SUBSCRIBE ON APPLE PODCASTS

Ready to listen? Make sure you have the appropriate podcast app installed on your mobile device to enjoy our latest episodes.

https://tinyurl.com/WINTODAYSHOW